Osteopathy for Children

Third edition

Elizabeth C. Hayden D.O.

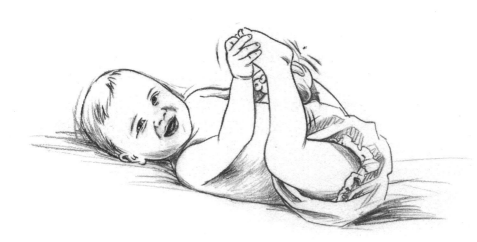

Written and published by Elizabeth C. Hayden D.O.
Illustrations by Angela Lumley and Geoff Jones.
Designed and produced by Viners Wood Associates, 01452 812813.
Printed in England by Biddles Limited, Guildford.

Further copies obtainable from:
Churchdown Osteopaths, 102 Chosen drive, Churchdown Gloucester GL3 2QU.

ISBN 0 9532542 0 8

Contents

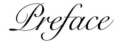

A personal experience of cranial osteopathy

Osteopathy is a philosophy of health not just a series of techniques applied to the body. This philosophy acknowledges that in health the body should be able to automatically adapt to different demands, and maintain itself in a state of balance and harmony. The body is always doing its best to maintain a state of balance, and can recover from or adapt to many traumatic events. However its resources for coping are not endless, and sometimes events occur that are too much for the body to correct without assistance. This is where osteopathy can help.

Symptoms?
Romilly was 11 months at the time, an energetic child with a quick smile. She was way ahead of the normal developmental milestones and was already walking around the shops with us! On the face of it all was fine. Unfortunately her physical feats surpassed her intellectual development. She was a danger to herself while awake and took little daytime sleep. At night she woke often, cried often, and repeatedly tapped her head against the cot. My wife was exhausted and I was close behind. We even felt guilty that, sometimes, we wished Romilly was less 'awake'; it seemed so ungrateful.

At a personal level I have benefited from osteopathy for many years, yet I probably wouldn't have thought of cranial osteopathy for Romilly. Luckily, my professional life revolves around avoiding back pain and preserving posture, particularly in children, (I am passionate about the way poor seating damages posture and damages our children's spines!). As if on cue a cranial osteopath telephoned to ask if she could run a children's cranial practice at one of my *Children's Seating Centres*. She felt our work was compatible and it seemed the ideal opportunity to see if anything was behind Romilly's behaviour pattern.

Cure?
Frankly we were delighted. The head tapping, early waking and poor sleep patterns all stopped. The osteopath treated Romilly for retained stress at the back of the skull. No wonder it was painful to crawl with the head

pulled back and it explained why standing was preferable. Chances are the head was uncomfortable when still.

I already knew that children's posture is important, and the osteopathy was a great place to go for falls and injuries in childhood. Now though I can understand why many parents have found cranial osteopathy to help their children.

As this book explains, early treatment leads to easier correction, so my feeling is that a visit to a cranial osteopath could become a natural part of a young baby's life.

David Newbound

David Newbound writes each month on children's environments in *Natural Parent*. He currently heads the Children's Working Party for the National Back Pain Association and runs two shops: Back in Action (posture correction for adults) and Children's Seating Centres (healthy children's furniture).

Introduction

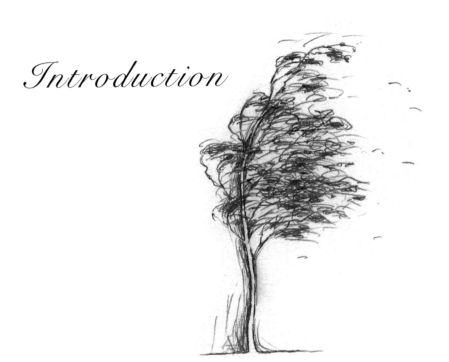

Why do children need to see an osteopath?

It is a common belief that children and babies should have no structural stresses and strains in their body, because they are so young and flexible. The reality is very different.

The birth of a baby is one of the most stressful events of its life. The baby is subjected to enormous forces as the uterus (or womb) pushes to expel the baby against the natural resistance of the birth canal. The baby has to turn and twist as it squeezes through the bony pelvis, on its short but highly stimulating and potentially stressful journey into the outside world.

The baby's head has the ability to mould and change shape in response to the stresses of a normal labour. The distortions in the head as a result of labour are usually released naturally afterwards. However there are many reasons why labour may be difficult and stressful for both mother and baby, as a result of which the baby may be unable to fully resolve the effects of birth. If birth stresses remain unresolved then the baby has to adapt to and accommodate these stresses and strains as he/she grows. This may cause the baby to either be physically uncomfortable and therefore unhappy, or to develop in an asymmetrical way.

If a baby's body becomes twisted or severely strained at birth, then the whole body will grow in a distorted way and every structure of the body will be required to cope with this distortion. The degree of distortion will relate to the severity of the original strain. This is similar to the way in which a tree growing with a prevailing wind on one side will grow crooked. The same is true of the human body.

Evidence of these distortions is readily seen in people's faces. Careful study of a face will often reveal signs of asymmetry. An easy way of demonstrating this is to place a small mirror in the centre of a photograph of a face, and view each half reflected as a whole (*see below*). Both reflected halves often look completely different. Asymmetry can also be seen in other areas of the body. Often one shoulder is held higher than the other, one side of the pelvis may be higher than the other, or one foot turned outwards more than the other.

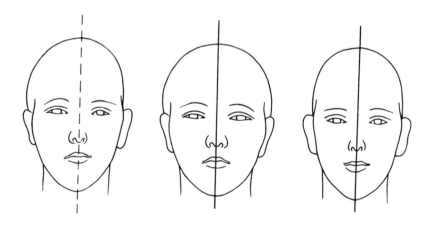

Unresolved birth stresses and the body's adaptations to them are at the root of many different problems both in childhood and right into adult life. These stresses can usually be treated very quickly after birth, but become progressively more difficult to eliminate the longer they have been present.

This book aims to give some background into the most common problems and their causes that we see in babies and children. It cannot be comprehensive since each child is unique.

What is osteopathy?

Osteopathy is a philosophy of health not just a series of techniques applied to the body. This philosophy acknowledges that in health the body should be able to automatically adapt to different demands, and maintain itself in a state of balance and harmony. The body is always doing its best to maintain a state of balance, and can recover from or adapt to many traumatic events. However its resources for coping are not endless, and sometimes events occur that are too much for the body to correct without assistance. This is where osteopathy can help.

Osteopaths diagnose and treat structural stresses and strains that may be interfering with health. Osteopathy is well known to be beneficial for aches and pains in the musculoskeletal structures of the body. Less well known is that it can also help an enormous variety of different symptoms and problems in babies, children and adults.

Osteopaths treat the whole person, not just the areas of the body causing symptoms. This is because the cause of a problem often has its origin in another part of the body. It is possible to have several people with exactly the same symptoms but each has a different reason for developing, and needs different treatment. It follows that no two osteopathic treatments are the same. Osteopaths are continually searching to understand and treat the underlying cause of a particular problem, rather than just treating the symptoms.

Many of the problems that osteopaths see in our patients, both in adults and children, have their origin in unresolved birth stresses. For this reason much of the information in this booklet is about the birth process, and the effects it can have on babies and children. Many osteopaths believe that all babies should be routinely checked by an osteopath after birth.

What does an osteopath do?

Following a careful diagnosis, a variety of carefully applied manipulative procedures and approaches are used to release areas of mechanical stress. Many of these techniques are extremely gentle and rarely painful. This allows the body to begin to express its full health potential.

In the few days following an osteopathic treatment, the body will make its own adjustments to the release of physical strains and stresses. The whole body benefits from this re-balancing process, and as a result patients often report an improvement in many aspects of health. This may include the relief of the original symptoms that took them to the osteopath in the

9

first place, as well as a variety of other things. Almost anything can improve with treatment, things as diverse as any physical pain, sleep patterns, energy levels, constipation, emotional wellbeing, immunity to illnesses etc.

Osteopaths treat using a variety of different methods

Osteopaths are probably best known for the traditional manipulative techniques that produce the characteristic 'click' of joints (loved by some and feared by others!). However there are many different ways an osteopath can achieve results, and it is a matter for individual osteopaths to decide which techniques or approaches they prefer and which work best for them.

Cranial osteopathy

One of the fastest growing areas of osteopathy is known as 'cranial osteopathy'. This is a very subtle and gentle approach to the treatment of the whole body (not just the head, as is implied from the name). Cranial osteopathy is not different to osteopathy, it simply recognises the importance of the subtle mechanics at work within the head, and their profound influence on the health of the whole body.

Many osteopaths have training in the cranial approach, but not all. It is a specialised field, and involves considerable postgraduate study.

Osteopaths do not like the term 'cranial osteopathy', since it does not accurately describe the approach, and there has been much debate within the profession over many years about this name. However, many members of the public are familiar with the term cranial osteopathy, and it seems that we are (reluctantly) stuck with it. Some osteopaths prefer the term 'paediatric osteopathy' to indicate a special interest in the treatment of children.

In general the approach to osteopathy outlined in this book is embraced by the cranial approach. The gentle nature of cranial treatment makes it particularly suitable for the treatment of children, but children may not be treated exclusively with 'cranial' techniques.

The osteopathic profession

In the past, regulation of osteopaths by a professional body was voluntary and there were several different Registers of Osteopaths. Anyone could call him or herself an osteopath with little or no training, and were not required to belong to any professional registering body. This was obviously a very confusing and potentially dangerous situation for members of the public wishing to find a qualified practitioner.

This situation changed with the Osteopaths Act 1993, which established a new body, the General Osteopathic Council (or GOsC), to bring the whole profession under statutory, rather than voluntary, self-regulation. The GOsC opened the statutory register in 1998, and the Act became fully enacted from May 2000. It is now a criminal offence for anyone to claim to be, or to practise as an osteopath unless he or she is a member of the statutory register. This is obviously an important safeguard to standards for the public.

Osteopathic training

Most osteopaths receive a 4 year full time training. Some Colleges of Osteopathy offer part time or extended pathway courses, lasting up to 6 years, which are helpful to mature students who need to work to support themselves whilst training.

Regardless of the way the training is structured, all osteopaths study both practical and theoretical subjects, including in depth study of anatomy, physiology, pathology, medicine, nutrition etc. This gives the student a sound knowledge of how the body works in health as well as in disease. There is also an extensive clinical training.

1

Pregnancy and the Developing Baby

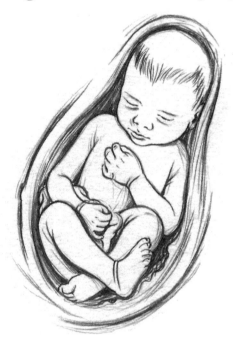

*W*hen a child visits an osteopath he/she has his own unique story to tell of his short life. He will have been influenced by an enormous number of factors, beginning with the health of his parents before birth, and including a wide range of physical, chemical, nutritional and emotional influences during his nine months (usually) in the womb. He has gradually developed into the person he is today. Osteopaths recognise that certain things happen during the child's life in the womb that can have an adverse effect on healthy growth and development. Some of the ongoing effects on the child of these early traumas can be reduced by appropriate osteopathic treatment, once the cause of their problem has been identified.

Life inside the uterus

From the moment of conception when the sperm meets and penetrates the egg, the newly formed embryo begins an incredibly rapid process of growth and development. In the first eight weeks it changes from a single cell into a recognisably human shape. By this stage all the major systems of the body have fully formed. The limbs including fingers and toes have formed, the brain, digestive system, and tiny lungs are present. The circulatory system has developed and the heart is beating. This incredibly rapid development of the embryo occurs even before the placenta has formed, and at this stage the embryo gets its nutrition from stored energy reserves in the egg. Much of this development occurs before the mother even knows that she is pregnant.

At approximately 12 weeks after fertilisation the placenta takes over in supplying nutrition to the baby from the mother's circulation. This is a common time for miscarriage due to the change in hormonal activity in the mother.

From 8 to 40 weeks the baby grows and matures in preparation for his entry into the world. During this time, the baby gradually becomes aware of his environment and learns to move and explore it.

The earliest of the senses to develop is hearing. The inner ear, the part contained within bone inside the skull, is fully formed and adult size by 23 weeks after fertilisation[1]. From this time the baby is able to hear sounds, and the brain begins learning to interpret them. Most mothers will know that their baby responds to sound during the pregnancy, perhaps by startling at loud noises, or becoming particularly active when a certain piece of music is played. After birth, a baby seems to recognise and may be soothed by music that he heard a lot whilst in the womb. The womb is a continually noisy place, with the constant rhythmical sound of the mother's heartbeat, intestinal gurgling, as well as slightly muffled sounds from outside. The baby usually recognises the familiar sound of his mother's voice soon after birth. It is not surprising that young babies relax better if there is some background noise rather than complete silence.

The developing baby is a unique individual right from the start, and aspects of his character are often evident even whilst still in the womb. Often the baby who is never still during pregnancy is also a very active baby after birth. Likewise a baby who moves little in the womb is more likely to be a placid baby after birth. It is this individuality that makes each child respond emotionally and physically in his or her own unique way to particular events during the pregnancy.

It is this individual response that is of interest to an osteopath in the treatment of a baby or child. The osteopath tries to gain an understanding of any physical and emotional stresses that have been experienced by a baby or child, including those during life in the uterus. Some of these events have very obvious effects on the baby, others are much more subtle, including barely perceptible effects on the quality or vitality of the body tissues. In treatment, recognition of the cause of poor vitality in a baby is of enormous value in helping to improve that health state.

Events during pregnancy that can affect the developing baby

Health of the Parents

To give their baby the best possible start in life, both parents need to be in a state of good health before the child is conceived. Poor health in either parent can undermine the vitality of a developing baby, which may then make it more difficult for the child to cope with subsequent traumas such as birth, or illness. Mothers who have conceived soon after coming off the pill are often low in certain vitamins, and it is thought that this may have an effect on the underlying health state of the developing baby.

Nausea and sickness

Nausea and sickness are very common during the first few weeks of pregnancy. The effects usually pass by 12-14 weeks. In some unfortunate mothers, the sickness may persist for much longer, even throughout the whole pregnancy. Long-term sickness and associated poor eating habits can have a detrimental effect on the available nutrition to the baby, and the baby may be small at birth. If the available nutrients are low at certain stages of development notably when the centres of the brain that control appetite are developing, it has been observed that the baby may be a voracious feeder later on. The effects of persistent deprivation of oxygen or nutrients during pregnancy can sometimes be palpated in the body tissues of the baby during osteopathic treatment.

Smoking

It is well known that smoking in either parent can reduce fertility. Mothers who smoke in pregnancy are more likely to have small babies, and evidence indicates that babies of parents who smoke are more likely to succumb to cot death in infancy. Later, the children of parents who smoke are more likely to suffer from respiratory problems such as asthma. The evidence is overwhelming that smoking by either or both parents is harmful to babies. The effects are often palpable osteopathically in the child, the tissues of the body have a characteristic unhealthy quality and they may be slower to respond to treatment.

Illness

An osteopath is interested in any illness suffered by the mother during pregnancy. In general the baby is unaffected by these illnesses, and even when a mother is quite seriously ill during pregnancy, the baby is usually born perfectly healthy. However certain illnesses at critical times can have some ongoing effect. The effect depends on the stage of development of the baby.

In the first few weeks, while the organs and systems of the body are still developing, the development of some part may be affected. An extreme example of this is German Measles (Rubella), which can interfere with the development of the ear and lead to deafness in the baby if it is contracted during the first three months of pregnancy. Fortunately this is now rare due to vaccinations against Rubella. Other acute illnesses (such as acute infections, either viral or bacterial) or long-term illness (such as diabetes) can have less dramatic effects on the baby.

After 12 weeks the foetus is fully formed, but is still very small. The rest of the pregnancy is devoted to growth and maturation of the various organs and organ systems, and the baby is then generally less seriously affected by illness in the mother. Any external influence strong enough to affect the developing baby is more likely to act as a check on its growth rate, rather than influencing the way structures are developing. The resultant baby may be perfectly normal, just behind average in reaching the normal developmental milestones.

In some cases a traumatic event or illness in the mother can have an effect on the baby that can be likened to driving a car with the brakes partly engaged. The car will work, but slower than normal. In a baby, normal development may be possible but at a slower rate. The baby or child falls progressively further behind in his/her development, perhaps being late in sitting, crawling, walking or talking. Later on, learning at school may be slow and difficult. Osteopathic treatment can sometimes be effective in 'unbinding the brakes', identifying and treating the relevant obstruction, thus allowing development to continue at a more normal rate.

Drugs

Drugs taken in pregnancy can affect the developing baby. An extreme example of this was Thalidomide, a drug used in the 1960s to help relieve sickness in pregnancy, and which caused limb deformities. It is advisable to avoid all unnecessary drugs during pregnancy if possible. Medical advice should be sought as to whether unavoidable drugs are known to have any effect on the baby.

Drugs like cocaine, LSD, heroine etc., directly affect the nervous system of the mother. They have the same effect on the nervous system of the child, and can delay development. Whilst these drugs are only taken by a small minority of the population, derivatives are commonly prescribed for a wide variety of conditions suffered by a larger percentage of the population (e.g. opium derivatives used in sedatives or strong painkillers such as morphine. Pethidine is also an opium-based painkiller). Their effects are sometimes palpable after birth by those people with the necessary skills and training.

Asthma in the mother

Mild asthma in pregnancy has no effect on the developing baby because mild asthma does not significantly reduce the oxygen in the mother's blood stream. Severe asthma over a long period of time, or sudden very acute attacks can temporarily deprive the baby for oxygen and leave a lasting effect.

▶ Case History

Robert was brought in for treatment at age 2¹/2 with signs of spasticity in his legs. He could walk, but his movements were slow and awkward, and he fell a great deal. There was no apparent cause from birth and the most obvious reason for Robert's disability was that his mother had experienced a severe asthma attack two thirds of the way through the pregnancy.

During osteopathic examination and treatment, a palpable level of shock and stress was felt in the normal delicate motion of the brain. It appeared that this was the result of the anoxia (lack of oxygen) caused by his mother's asthma attack. Its effect was twofold, firstly the short lived effect of the lack of oxygen, and secondly an ongoing hindrance to the development of Robert's brain in the area that controlled his legs, which added to the original damage. Treatment was administered to release the shock still present in the brain, to relax the tension in his leg muscles and help the developing posture.

17

▶ **Comment**

It is obviously not possible to turn back the clock, and repair any brain damage caused by anoxia, but treatment can help to reduce long-term effects, and enable the child to develop to his/her fullest potential.

The placenta

In the womb the baby needs a steady and maintained supply of nutrients and oxygen from the mother. These reach the baby through the placenta, which has to be functioning well for optimum growth. Any reduction in the supply of nutrients reaching the baby via the placenta can lead to a slowed rate of growth of the baby. The placenta also acts as a filter to help keep unwanted substances out of the baby's blood stream.

The placenta is always examined in detail after birth. This is partly to ensure that the uterus has expelled it all, and also to assess its state of health. In a post mature infant, i.e. one that has gone past the due delivery date, the placenta can lose some of its efficiency, and become 'gritty' or fragmented. This is the reason that mothers who have not delivered two weeks after their due date are checked carefully, as signs of distress in the baby may be due to degeneration of the placenta.

Occasionally the placenta may lose its efficiency early, which deprives the baby of essential oxygen and nutrition. This can delay growth towards the end of pregnancy, and even damage the baby if the deprivation has been prolonged or severe.

Accidents and trauma to the mother

Early in pregnancy the baby is well protected in the uterus by its fluid environment, and also by the bony pelvis surrounding it.

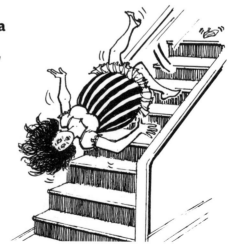

From mid pregnancy onwards, the baby is growing in size and does not have the same amount of fluid and tissue protection around it. If the mother has an accident such as a fall or impact in the pelvic or abdominal region, the baby may be vulnerable to physical injury or shock. This may need to be treated after birth.

Road traffic accidents can be particularly traumatic to the baby in the last three months of pregnancy, because by this stage the baby takes up most of the space in the mother's abdomen and pelvis, and is more likely to come into direct contact with bony structures. In addition, the mother's shape necessitates the seat belt passing directly over the uterus and baby. Not only is the baby vulnerable to having his head bumped against the bony pelvis, but also the body can be compressed by the seat belt.

▶ **Case History**
Baby Sarah was brought into the practice for treatment when she was four months old. She was very fretful and irritable and wouldn't settle or go to sleep easily. The pregnancy had been good, the birth uncomplicated and an average length of 6-8 hours long. There seemed no obvious reason why Sarah should be so unsettled. Her mother then revealed that she had fallen downstairs on her bottom when 8 months pregnant.

When Sarah was examined there was a localised area of compression in the region of the occiput at the back of her head, which was creating tension in all the tissues around it. This was not recognisable as the sort of compression received during birth, and was thought to have been caused by the back of her head coming into contact with her mother's pelvis during the fall.

When the effects were released Sarah lost her irritability and rapidly settled into a much happier baby.

Moulding during pregnancy

Moulding is the name given to the change in shape of the baby's head as it descends through the mother's pelvis during delivery. The process of moulding often begins during late pregnancy.

A baby growing in the uterus, bathed in the amniotic fluid surrounding it, should normally be relatively free of external pressures. However, the body tissues of the developing baby are very soft, and will distort if pressure is maintained on any one part. As the baby grows it takes up a position that is most comfortable within the uterus. This will naturally be a position with the least amount of maintained pressure on any one part.

Normally this is with the head down in the mother's pelvis.

If the baby is particularly cramped in the uterus as with a very large baby, a small mother, a small amount of amniotic fluid, or with twins, then parts of the baby may be subjected to maintained pressure. This may cause those parts to grow in a distorted manner, and can set up strain patterns that are palpable by an osteopath after birth. Babies who sit in the breech position in the uterus often have their arms and legs in funny positions, and usually have their head pressed tight up under the mother's ribs. This is uncomfortable for both mother and baby, and will often cause moulding in the head as it grows. Distorted heads can often be improved by osteopathic treatment after birth, although it is not always possible to fully resolve asymmetries.

Moulding begun in the uterus is increased during the birth process. This is described in Chapter 3. After birth, when the baby is free of the confined space of the uterus, some of these moulding patterns are corrected at the same time as the birth moulding is released. In other cases the moulding begun in the uterus does not release and birth moulding is added to it, contributing to the effects on the baby described later.

Emotional stress

Babies are very sensitive to emotional stress experienced by the mother during pregnancy, particularly when it is affecting her own emotional security as a prospective mother. Maternal stresses that have a particular effect are undue anxiety for the health of the baby, difficulties in her relationship with her partner, family bereavement or anything causing insecurity in the home, such as building work or a house move.

This does not mean that every time a mother is feeling stressed she is harming her baby, because babies are able to deal with short-lived stresses. It is when stress levels are raised over a long period of time that the effects are detrimental to the baby.

Stress in the mother causes the release of adrenaline into her bloodstream, which also passes to the baby. The baby's own adrenaline level is thus temporarily raised. If this situation persists over a long period of time, the raised adrenaline level may gradually become the normal level for the baby. Subsequently his ability to cope with stress is working from a pre-set higher level, and as a result he has less reserves to cope with stressful situations than he might otherwise have done.

This may manifest as a level of tension or anxiety in the baby after birth. The baby may be insecure and clingy, and is often oversensitive to noise and light. Babies are more likely to suffer from infantile colic in the early months of life if the mother has suffered from stress in pregnancy[2].

It also interesting to observe that babies and children may show a particular intolerance to the specific type of stress that their mother was subjected to in pregnancy, for example disruption in the home.

▶ Case History

Baby Thomas, age 2 months, could be heard very clearly in the waiting room! He was constantly crying, and would only be held by his mother. He was fretful and his little fists were always tightly clenched. He was over-sensitive, jumped at the slightest noises and did not like bright lights. Thomas' parents were distraught and did not know what to do to pacify him.

The birth had been easy and there was not enough retained moulding present around the head for the birth to be considered the cause of his distress. However, Thomas felt extremely tense, in all his body tissues.

When questioned closely it became apparent that Thomas' mother had suffered several miscarriages before conceiving Thomas. She started the pregnancy being worried and with the threatened miscarriage early on, she became fearful that Thomas would be lost as well.

During osteopathic examination and treatment, it was felt that the anxiety suffered by Thomas' mother during pregnancy had led to him being tense and over-reactive. Thomas was treated using appropriate gentle manipulative treatment to release his tension, and to attempt to reduce his 'pre-set level' of stress. Thomas gradually became more relaxed, and his parents could then start to enjoy the baby that they had waited so long to have.

2

Osteopathy during Pregnancy

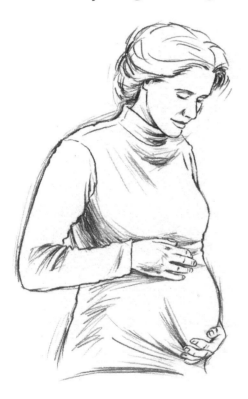

$\mathscr{P}$ regnancy is a very physical experience. The mother has to gradually adapt to carrying up to 20lb of baby, waters and placenta during the pregnancy – the equivalent of almost 10 bags of sugar! The whole body has to adapt to carrying this large mass, and it can impose physical strain on all the organs and tissues around it.

A mother who is physically fit at the start of pregnancy will generally have an easier and more comfortable time both during the pregnancy and in the labour. Being physically fit does not just mean having well exercised muscles and feeling well. What an osteopath means by describing someone as fit for pregnancy is that the body is free of unnecessary tensions and strains that may compromise the pregnancy, and is ready and able to adapt to the various physical demands of pregnancy and labour.

Our bodies are rarely perfect, and may be affected by strains and stresses in a way that is not always noticeable. These stresses are accumulated throughout life, starting with our own birth, falls and accidents, and other physical or emotional trauma. We are often completely unaware that these stresses are present because the body is very good at adapting and compensating, enabling us to continue our daily lives with no aches, pain or other symptoms. However if the body is unable to fully compensate then we may suffer symptoms such as musculoskeletal aches and pains including headache, or a wide variety of symptoms including general fatigue.

Many people suffer some sort of regular physical discomfort, often considered to be a normal and inevitable part of life, and pregnancy in particular. Many of these discomforts can be alleviated with osteopathic treatment. Whilst some women are fit, healthy and full of energy throughout pregnancy, the majority of women suffer various discomforts. For some, pregnancy is a very difficult time.

Pregnancy is a unique event for a mother's body. Enormous physical, chemical and emotional changes take place over a relatively short period of time. The baby literally takes over, and the mother has to adapt. Mothers often say that it is like being on a runaway train, and feel that they have no control over the dramatic changes taking place in their body during the pregnancy and birth.

Osteopathy during and after pregnancy

Osteopathic treatment can be beneficial during the pregnancy in several ways:
- Easing some of the physical discomforts of pregnancy
- In some cases helping stabilise a threatened miscarriage
- Preparing the mother's body for the demands of labour
- Helping recovery afterwards from both the pregnancy and delivery (see chapter 6)

An osteopathic examination before becoming pregnant or during early pregnancy can help to identify physical limitations and strains in the mother's body, which may interfere with the developing pregnancy and ultimately the labour and delivery. The earlier that treatment can start the better. Ideally it should be a part of preparation for pregnancy, and begin before conception. Osteopathy in first few months of pregnancy is beneficial in releasing longstanding physical strains and stresses from the body, as well as relieving any physical discomforts.

As the pregnancy progresses and the mother's body is challenged to adapt to the chemical and increasing physical changes, there is a subtle change that alters the way the body responds to osteopathic treatment. A strong overriding protective mechanism comes into play, which places the current demand for the protection of the unborn baby before any requirements of addressing longstanding physical strain. Baby comes first! As a result osteopathic treatment becomes more symptomatic, being beneficial in making pregnancy more comfortable and helping to prepare for labour, but with less work possible on pre-existing strains within the mother.

Postural changes during pregnancy

As the uterus grows the mother's body has to cope with the extra weight, and also to accommodate the increased size and shape of the uterus or womb. There are many more changes taking place than the visibly obvious protruding of the abdomen.

In the first few weeks there is a dramatic increase in blood flow to the uterus. This can give rise to bloating or heaviness in the pelvis similar to that experienced by many women just before a period. In the first 12 weeks the uterus is contained deep within the bony pelvis, and as it expands it can cause some pressure on the bladder, increasing the frequency with which the bladder needs to be emptied.

Between 12 and 16 weeks the top of the uterus called the 'fundus' begins to rise up into the abdomen. This usually eases discomfort within the pelvis but occasionally causes back pain due to the change in tension of the ligaments supporting the uterus, and their effect on the pelvis and lower spine.

During the middle three months of the pregnancy, the increasing size of the uterus begins to demand postural adaptation in the mother. Normally the abdominal muscles support the uterus and help contain it within the abdomen so that the stomach remains fairly flat at this stage. There is a tendency for a drag to be imposed on the membranes in the front of the body as the uterus enlarges. This can cause a variety of problems including tension across the shoulders, headache, or blocked nasal sinuses due to the pull of the enlarging uterus dragging on the viscera or organs of the chest and throat, and hence onto the face and base of the skull.

From about 30 weeks, the baby takes up most of the available space within the abdomen, and begins to crowd the lower part of the rib cage. The diaphragm is pushed higher up into the thorax or chest and the lower ribs flare out to help increase the available space.

In the final stages of pregnancy when any available internal space has been taken up, the only way that the uterus can enlarge is forwards and the size of the bulge increases dramatically. The increased weight at the front has to be balanced by the mother's shoulders and thorax moving backwards. This causes changes in the body's centre of gravity and shape of the spine. There may be an increase in the hollow of the lower back due to the weight of the uterus and baby dragging on the spine from the front. This is not good for the spine, and is one cause of backache in pregnancy. Poor posture may also cause neck ache, headaches, aching legs and undue fatigue.

Different shaped bumps!

There is an enormous variation in the shape of pregnant women. This can be for a variety of reasons, mostly to do with the height and abdominal muscle tone of the mother. The amount of amniotic fluid around the baby will also influence the size of the bump.

In shorter women there is less space within the abdomen for the baby, so the bump tends to protrude more. A tall woman can accommodate even a quite large baby within the abdomen without the bump appearing unduly large.

The tone of the abdominal muscles makes a difference to the size of the bump. Strong muscles will keep the baby contained better than weak ones. This is the reason that women tend to have a smaller bump in the first pregnancy when the muscles have not been stretched before, than in subsequent pregnancies. Good tone in the abdominal muscles helps to support the spine, helps prevent a very sway-backed posture from developing, and reduces backache.

If the diaphragm is unduly tense then the lower ribs may not be able to spread. This may be due to imbalances in spinal mechanics, physical strains or emotional stress in the mother. In this case the bump is carried all at the front, and may appear very large.

Good posture

The position of the baby will make a difference to the size and shape of the bump. For example the bump is more likely to be large and protruding if the baby is lying in the posterior or back to back position.

Self help tips for keeping fit during pregnancy

- Pregnancy is not a good time to start doing strenuous exercise if you are not used to it, but you should try to keep as active as possible in order to maintain good muscle tone. Swimming and walking can be continued throughout the pregnancy. Swimming is particularly good in the latter stages, because the water helps to support the weight of the baby.
- Yoga relaxation and gentle stretching exercises can be very beneficial throughout pregnancy.
- When walking or standing, stand tall pushing your head upwards but without sticking your chin out, as if suspended from the ceiling by a string. This can help to reduce the sway-backed posture.
- Avoid standing still for long periods.

Position of the baby

As the baby grows during the pregnancy there is progressively less space for him/her to move about and change positions. The baby finds his/her preferred position, and the mother's posture has to accommodate. If this conflicts with her own musculoskeletal demands, it may cause undue aches and pains. This is the reason that one pregnancy may be much more uncomfortable to carry than another.

The baby generally settles in a head downward position and facing backwards. This puts him/her in the most advantageous position for passing through the birth canal during labour.

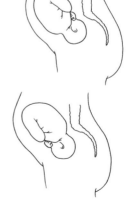

Sometimes the baby comes to lie in a 'back to back' or facing forward position. In this case kicking movements are all felt in the front, and the mother may suffer considerable backache due to the pressure of the baby's spine against her own.

The baby may lie in a breech position, or bottom downward. In this case the baby's head may be wedged firmly up under the mother's rib cage. This can be very uncomfortable for both mother and baby, causing bruising to the mother's ribs and distortion or moulding of the baby's head.

Later in pregnancy as the baby's head drops down into the pelvis and imparts pressure on the soft tissues of the pelvis. This can cause symptoms as diverse as pressure on the bladder that makes the mother empty her bladder more frequently, local pain in the lower back or pelvis, or nerve pain down one leg if the pressure is on a nerve.

In most cases osteopathic treatment to ensure that the pelvis and uterus are correctly balanced and aligned can help with discomforts caused by the baby's position, and can often help the baby turn into a better position.

Self-help tips to encourage the baby to lie correctly
As labour is likely to be more difficult if the baby is not lying correctly, it is worth trying to help him/her to move into a better position.
So, what can you do to help yourself during the pregnancy?
- Try to keep as active as possible throughout the pregnancy, and maintain good posture at all times. To help your posture, 'stand and walk tall' as if suspended by a piece of string from the top of your head. Try not to allow your lower back to drop into a very hollow shape.
- Sitting slouched in soft chairs encourages the baby to turn into the back to back position. Where possible, sit with your bottom well back in the chair and the lower back supported. Better still, sitting on a foam wedge or on a chair that has a seat that tilts forward, actively encourages the baby to lie correctly.
- If your baby is lying in either a breech or back to back position, then spending some time each day in an 'all fours' position (or crawling) can help him/her to turn.

The discomforts of pregnancy

Nausea and vomiting
During the first 12–16 weeks it is common for women to suffer nausea and vomiting and feel excessively tired. Osteopathy can sometimes be of help in restoring a feeling of well-being by releasing debilitating physical strains and restoring musculoskeletal harmony and balance. Treatment to improve the circulation to and from the liver can help with nausea.

Heart burn

During pregnancy the lower ribs and broad muscular sheet of the diaphragm gradually spread to increase the size of the abdominal cavity. This can place strain on the sphincter at the top of the stomach, which is formed by a loop of muscle from the diaphragm curling around the lower end of the oesophagus. This sphincter normally keeps all the stomach contents tightly inside, but if stretched or distorted it may allow small amounts of its acidic contents to leak back up into the oesophagus. This causes the classic burning sensation of heartburn. Osteopathic treatment can often help to alleviate heartburn by relaxing tension in the diaphragm, thus helping it to change shape without any undue stretch on any part, so helping the sphincter to function better.

Breathing difficulties

The increasing size of the abdomen, and the resulting change of shape of the lower ribs and diaphragm that has been described reduces the available volume of the lungs. This may cause some breathlessness, particularly when lying down.

Osteopathic treatment can improve function of the whole rib cage and enable full use of its available capacity. This also helps the lymphatic system to function efficiently, which in turn assists the immune system of the body.

Varicose veins and haemorrhoids

Varicose veins in the legs and haemorrhoids are common in pregnancy. There are two main reasons for these to develop. In part they are a side effect of the action of the hormones that soften ligaments during pregnancy. These hormones do not act solely on ligaments, but also on all connective tissues in the body, including the veins. Veins that have been softened by hormonal action are more liable to stretch when under pressure.

Increased pressure within veins may be caused by any restriction in the return of venous blood to the heart. The diaphragm has to make considerable changes to its shape as it adapts to accommodate the growing uterus. In some cases this creates tension that can restrict the passage of venous blood from the lower half of the body back to the heart, and cause a slight increase of pressure in the venous system below the diaphragm.

The increasing size of the baby within the uterus may cause a slight increase of pressure on veins within the pelvis. This can either impose pressure on the veins of the rectum causing haemorrhoids, or restrict venous return from one or both legs, making them vulnerable to varicosities.

Self-help tips for prevention of varicose veins and haemorrhoids

- Walking is beneficial, but standing still for long periods should be avoided. Regular contraction of the calf muscles during walking helps to pump blood uphill through the veins of the legs back to the pelvis. It follows that plenty of walking is helpful, but standing still for long periods so that the calf muscles are not used is not advisable.
- Avoid sitting with the legs crossed, as this restricts venous return.
- Sit with the feet elevated whenever possible.
- Use a rocking chair if possible, to encourage gentle activity in the muscles of the legs and help stimulate venous drainage.
- Support tights can be helpful if signs of varicose veins appear, or if the legs are very achy.
- Osteopathic treatment to release tension in the pelvis and diaphragm regions is helpful in the prevention of varicose veins and haemorrhoids.

Aches and pains

If the mother had a back problem before becoming pregnant, or has suffered significant trauma to her back, neck, head or pelvis at any time in her life, then it may be very difficult for her body to make the necessary postural adjustments. As the spine struggles within its pre-existing limitations to accommodate the size and weight of the uterus, undue strain can be placed on all or part of the spine. As a result the muscles have to work harder to support the spine so that more energy is used for everyday activities. This may cause symptoms as diverse as back or neck ache or pain, numbness or 'pins and needles' in the arms or legs due to nerve irritation, headaches or undue fatigue.

An osteopath can identify regions of the spine that may be moving too much and are thus vulnerable to over-strain, or areas that are stiff and unable to yield to allow the posture to gradually adapt to the changing size and weight of the uterus. Treatment to harmonise the mobility throughout the spine allows the spine to find a balanced position and shape that can be maintained with a minimum of muscle tension. This is of course more comfortable as well.

The ligaments supporting the uterus undergo an enormous increase in thickness and length during pregnancy, and can cause pain and aching in the groins and lower abdomen. On occasions the uterus can become slightly twisted, which puts extra load on its ligaments. This can cause discomfort to the mother, and affect the position of the baby.

Specific osteopathic treatment can help release tension in the muscles of the pelvis and the ligaments supporting the uterus, and balance the relationship between the main pelvic bones and sacrum or tailbone. This relieves any strain in the joints and soft tissues of the pelvis and improves the general circulation within the pelvis and lower limbs.

Pubic symphysis pain

The pubic symphysis is the tough ligamentous junction at the front of the pelvis that joins the two halves of the pelvis together. Pain is often felt in this area during late pregnancy. The pain is caused partly by the normal softening of ligaments in pregnancy and partly from the pressure of the baby's head inside the pelvis. The pain can be quite intense, and may limit the amount of walking possible in the later stages of pregnancy. Osteopathic treatment may be of some help at this time, as may the wearing of a maternity corset to help support the pelvis and weight of the uterus.

The pubic symphysis can also suffer damage during childbirth if it is overstretched, causing a condition called *diastasis symphysis pubis*. In most cases this settles within a few weeks of birth, but in a minority it persists and mothers can suffer great pain for months after the birth. Any history of *diastasis symphysis pubis* leaves the area vulnerable to more strain in subsequent pregnancies.

Osteopathic treatment is extremely effective at correcting any positional displacement in the pubic symphysis after delivery, and re-balancing the ligaments. This allows the over-stretched ligaments of the pubic symphysis to gradually recover and can help to prevent much of the ongoing suffering that this condition causes.

Miscarriage

Miscarriage can be very distressing. It is relatively common, and there are many reasons for it to happen. One reason may be that it is the body's way of removing a damaged or malformed baby. In some cases the cause may be a hormonal imbalance in the mother. The baby is commonly miscarried at around 12 weeks when the placenta begins to take over the nutrition of the baby, which is a time of changes in the balance of hormones within the body.

Miscarriage is more common in first pregnancies. One theory to explain this is that the mother's hormones may not have started working sufficiently to support the pregnancy. Often the first pregnancy that miscarries 'kick starts' the hormonal system and the next pregnancy is carried to full term with no problem.

Some women suffer repeated miscarriage, often at the same stage of pregnancy each time. It is logical to assume that there must be some reason why this occurs. The cause may be hormonal, and progesterone supplements in the first few weeks have been found to help some women. However, there are many reasons for miscarriage.

Osteopathy can sometimes help to settle down a threatened miscarriage. Treatment is aimed at any area of the body where there is a mechanical imbalance. Particular attention is directed at relaxing the uterus which often feels very irritable as it is beginning to contract. Osteopathy will not prevent and inevitable miscarriage, or if there is a chemical or hormonal reason for miscarriage occurring. But for some women, it definitely works.

In some cases there are physical problems that make it difficult for a pregnancy to carry beyond a certain stage. The mother's body may be physically unable to support the weight of the baby, fluids, placenta and uterus, resulting in a 'fatigue based' miscarriage often later in the pregnancy. This may be caused by physical strains in the pelvis from past falls or accidents, or other injuries that limit the ability of the mother's body to adapt to the pregnancy. Osteopathic treatment can often help to settle the pregnancy and carry it through to a successful conclusion.

Another area of the body that can be important in the treatment of recurrent miscarriage is the face. This is an area that commonly carries effects of past trauma such as falls or blows to the face, or dental treatment such as orthodontics or wisdom tooth extractions. Tension in the face restricts the fascias or membranes down the front of the body to the pelvis, limiting the ability of the abdominal and pelvic tissues to accommodate the expanding uterus.

Physical distortion in the region of the pituitary gland in the head can sometimes interfere with the hormonal balance of the body, whether pregnant or not. Osteopathic treatment to reduce this physical strain may help hormonal balance in the body.

Preparation for labour

An important part of preparation for childbirth is to ensure that the mother's pelvis is structurally balanced and able to allow the passage of the baby down the birth canal. The baby's head is a tight fit within the pelvis, and every bit of extra space that can be gained is helpful. The size of the pelvic outlet can increase by as much as 30% during labour in a healthy pelvis, by a combination of the following:

- Secretion of hormones during the pregnancy that soften the ligaments and make them more able to stretch during labour.
- The two pelvic bones and the sacrum that make up the pelvis need to be able to separate slightly during labour to create more space for the baby to pass through. The coccyx moves backwards by about 30° in a normal labour to make way for the passage of the baby's head.
- The muscles of the pelvis also need to be able to relax fully to allow the baby to pass through.

Trauma to the pelvic bones, coccyx or sacrum at any time in a mother's life can leave increased tension in muscles and strain within ligaments and bones of the pelvis. This can limit the ability of the bones to separate and move out of the way during labour, and thus limit the size of the pelvic outlet. Osteopathic treatment is extremely effective at releasing old strains within the pelvis, thus giving the best chance of an easy and uncomplicated labour.

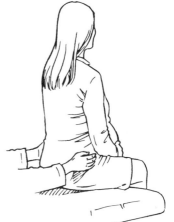

3

Adaptation of the Baby to the birth process

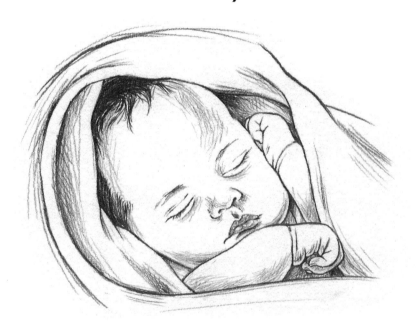

*I*n this chapter we look at the way the baby accommodates the intense pressures and distortions that are required during the birth process.

Structure of the skull

Contrary to common belief the skull is not a solid bony container, but is formed from 22 separate bones. In an adult skull these are all intricately jointed in such a way that they allow a very slight movement, or shape change of the whole container. This accommodates a subtle rhythmic movement of the brain inside.

An infant skull is required to have considerable flexibility to enable it to mould and pass through the birth canal, but it also needs to protect the delicate brain inside. It is cleverly structured so that it can perform both of these functions. At birth the bones are only partially formed, and the skull is more like a membranous bag with bony stiffening within it. The bones are strongest in the areas that take maximum compression during birth, and where they surround the most vulnerable parts of the brain. In other areas of the head the bones are much more malleable, and can distort under load without damage to the underlying structures. This intricate adaptation of the bones of the head provides good protection for the brain during a normal birth.

Development of the skull bones

In order to understand a how and why the baby's head moulds in labour, it is necessary to go back a little to the way the baby develops in the uterus.

In the early days of life, the baby is no more than a fluid filled mass of cells. Gradually different structures form and take shape. As the baby grows, the early skeleton begins to develop and gradually bones are formed, a process known as ossification.

Some bones (eg. the bones of the arms and legs) develop an outline of the adult bone made of

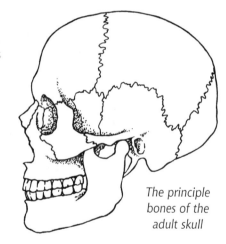

The principle bones of the adult skull

cartilage, which is like the flexible outer ear or the nose. These then gradually turn into more rigid bone – a process that is not completed until the age of 25 years. This is called cartilaginous ossification.

Other bones develop within a membrane, which gradually has bone cells laid down in it to stiffen it. This remains extremely flexible during its formation, and is the type of bone found in the top of the skull. This is called membranous ossification.

The baby's skull has both types of bone in it, that which forms from a cartilage 'proforma', and that which forms within a membrane. Cartilage is formed in the bones of the base (or floor) of the skull adjacent to the most delicate parts of the brain, to provide strength and protection from a very early stage of development. The bones of the vault of the skull – which is most of the head above the eyes and covered with hair, are formed from membrane (membranous ossification) which gives them maximum flexibility to accommodate growth of the brain, and also to adapt to the stresses of birth by allowing moulding.

After 40 weeks of pregnancy, the baby is ready to be born, and its skull is perfectly prepared for the adaptations necessary for a normally presented delivery. Simply stated, the baby's skull at birth is a bit like a balloon with stiffening plates in it, mounted on a more rigid but still slightly flexible base.

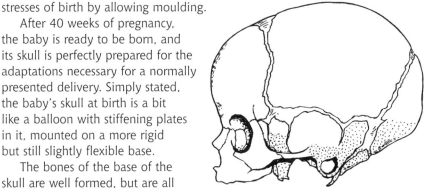

Baby's skull from the side

☐ *Bone ossified in membrane*

▦ *Bone ossified from cartilage*

The bones of the base of the skull are well formed, but are all made up partly of bone and partly of cartilage. The bony parts are relatively stiff and protect the brain, while the cartilage provides a kind of internal hinging which allows the bone to distort and bend, without breaking. In addition, in a baby all bones are relatively soft and can bend under load. This is similar to the flexibility of young growth on a tree that can bend under load, and spring back to the original shape after the load or strain is removed.

A particularly interesting bone is the occiput – the bone at the back of the head. The occiput contains a large hole for the spinal cord to exit from the skull. This bone is in four parts at birth that are joined by

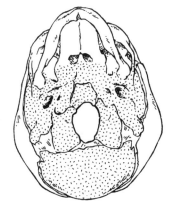

Baby's skull from underneath

cartilaginous 'hinges', allowing a complex shape change during the birth process, whilst still providing good protection to the spinal cord.

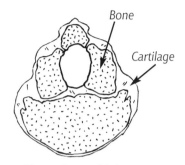

The bones of the vault (top of the head) are little more than stiffening plates in the membranes, and allow enormous shape changes while still protecting the delicate brain inside. They can overlap each other during birth to reduce the overall size of the head.

The occiput at birth

Moulding of the baby's head during labour

During normal labour the infant's head is subjected to very large compressive forces. These cause the head to undergo a process of moulding, in which the soft bones of the skull overlap, bend and warp. This reduces the size of the head and facilitates its passage through the birth canal.

While the cervix is dilating during the first stage of labour, the baby's head is pushed strongly into the cervix with each contraction. This helps the cervix to dilate, but also places the head under considerable compression. If the waters are intact, the bag of fluid cushions the baby's head within the cervix and distributes the force of contractions more evenly over the whole of the body of the baby. If the waters have already broken, then the head is no longer cushioned and undergoes more compression, which increases the amount of moulding.

During the second stage of labour, the pushing efforts of the mother combined with strong uterine contraction propel the baby downward in the pelvis. At the same time the baby's head has to twist and turn as it passes through the pelvis, with considerable resistance from the birth canal.

The forces imposed on the head result in distortion of the bones of the skull, and as a result some babies end up with extremely odd shaped heads when they are born.

The top of the neck, where the neck joins the skull, is a common area for compression, distortion and twisting to be found after birth. This is the area where the force of the uterine contractions pushing down on the baby's body, down the long axis of the spine, is met by resistance of the head in the cervix.

As already stated, the vault bones which form most of the head under the hair are flexible and able to overlap and distort with ease, and also able to return to normal after labour relatively easily. The stiffer bones of the base of the skull take more pressure to distort, and do not return to normal as easily after birth. It is the distortion in the bones of the base of the skull that cause many of the problems that osteopaths see in babies, children and adults. If distortion here is not corrected before the bone fully forms, at about one year old, than asymmetry is present for life. It is not only the head that undergoes compression and distortion during birth. The whole of the baby's body can become twisted, compressed and distorted as a result of the forces of labour. For example, asymmetrical forces during labour can distort the pelvis and spine, and in bigger babies the shoulders can become lodged within the pelvis and vulnerable to strain. Osteopaths always check the whole body of a baby during treatment, and take care to release stresses throughout the body.

The normal unmoulding process

After delivery the skull begins to re-expand and un-mould to return to its normal shape, assisted by the baby crying, suckling and yawning. The head is seen to gradually lose much of the moulding pattern during the first ten days of life. The majority of this shape-change arises from the soft bones of the vault re-expanding from their overlapped and squashed positions.

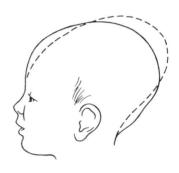

Far more difficult for the baby to release are the distortions in the stiffer bones of the cranial base. If the distortions remain within these bones, then as the bone continues to mature and the cartilage is replaced by harder bone, the warping within the bone becomes a permanent asymmetry. The bone can be left with a permanent feeling of strain held within its own structure. This strain can be transmitted to the delicate and pain sensitive meninges that surround the brain and stabilise it within its bony casing. This can have an effect on the brain itself, and in particular some of the cranial nerves as they exit from holes within and between the bones, and lead to many of the symptoms such as difficulties in suckling, and digesting food that are described in Chapter 5.

If birth has been particularly difficult or the baby has become stuck, larger forces are involved and the distortions are greater. It becomes even more difficult for the baby to release the retained distortions, resulting in more severe retained moulding compressions.

There is usually a gradual reduction in the moulding of the baby's head during the first ten days of life. During this time, the suckling action involved in breastfeeding acts as a powerful pump to assist the unmoulding process, aided by crying and yawning. After this, there is usually little unaided unmoulding of the head. The easier suckling action of bottlefeeding is less effective at helping the skull to re-expand after birth.

Many babies have odd shaped heads, which is invariably due to moulding during pregnancy or retained compression from birth. However, even in babies with an apparently good head shape, some quite marked strains can remain. As the child grows, any asymmetry becomes less obvious as it is covered by hair, but the stresses are still present. Untreated, retained birth compression remains present throughout life – try looking carefully at adult heads and faces and notice signs of asymmetry.

Some baby's heads show little sign of asymmetry after birth, but as they grow in the first six months, asymmetry becomes more obvious. This is because the areas of retained compression from birth are unable to grow freely, and so the compressed areas remain small compared with the 'free areas', and the asymmetry becomes exaggerated.

Osteopaths diagnose specific areas of retained distortion and compression in the bones of the head and use very careful, specific and accurately applied techniques to help guide the bones to a more comfortable balance. The younger that this is done the better, before the bones are fully developed so that any asymmetry is reduced as far as possible.

Retained moulding

Retained moulding from birth causes a very wide variety of problems in the baby. The effects are very individual, and some babies cope better than others. In some cases even quite severe moulding strains may cause no apparent problem as a young baby, but may predispose the child to other problems as they grow up – such as headaches, or an inability to cope well with future trauma. The effects of retained moulding are discussed in chapter 5.

4

Labour

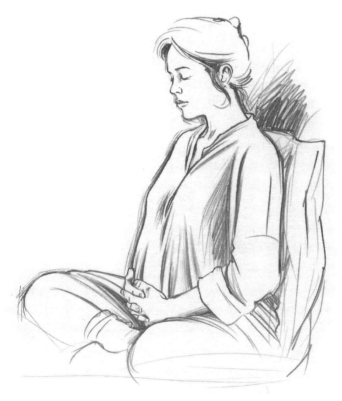

There are certain events during labour, and situations that may be present before labour starts (such as pre-existing strains in the mothers pelvis), that can cause greater than normal moulding in the babies head, or reduce his/her ability to release this moulding unassisted after birth. These things are of particular interest to an osteopath taking a case history of a baby or child.

A variety of different things that can influence normal and retained moulding in a baby are discussed in this chapter:

Limitation in the mother's pelvis

The pelvis is made up of three bones, the two innominate (or pelvic) bones, and the sacrum (or tailbone) between.

To help the passage of the head the three bones of the pelvis separate slightly during labour, both by stretching of the ligaments and by the individual bones tilting slightly.

The shape of the mother's pelvis may have been influenced in its development by stresses imposed on it. For example, if she was born as a breech delivery herself, then her sacrum and pelvis may have been subjected to enormous stresses during her birth, which can alter the shape as it develops. The sacrum and pelvis do not fully turn into bone until the mid twenties, before this they still have parts that are made of cartilage which is softer and more vulnerable to shape distortions if subjected to trauma. Accidents such as falls on the bottom while the sacrum and pelvis are still growing can have great influences on altering the shape of the bones as they grow. Later in life trauma to the pelvic area such as falls on the sacrum, coccyx, or hips, and some types of whiplash injuries can limit the ability of one or more of the parts to separate to its fullest extent during labour.

Stresses or shape distortions within the pelvis can restrict the ease of descent of the baby's head during the second stage of labour, and result in specific areas of compression in the infant skull. There is also increased likelihood that forceps or ventouse may be needed to assist delivery, which can add further moulding pressures on the baby's head.

Mothers who have structural difficulties in the pelvic area often suffer from backache during pregnancy. Osteopathic treatment before and during pregnancy can help to relieve backache of pregnancy, and assist in releasing some of the stresses in the pelvis to make it easier for the pelvis to expand during labour. This is obviously beneficial for both mother and baby.

Duration of labour

The length of labour can have a great influence on the amount of compression that the baby's head is subjected to, and also the subsequent amount of moulding.

Slow labour

A labour that is very long (over 15 hours) exposes the baby's head to large compressive forces for an extended period of time. This can be traumatic and the amount of moulding in the head is often extreme. However, some babies cope very well with a long, slow and controlled labour, and do not have significant retained moulding afterwards.

Rapid labour

A very rapid labour (less than 6 hours) can also be very stressful for the baby in a different way to a slow labour. Contractions are usually intense from the start, generating large compressive forces. The baby's head does not have time to mould gently and reduce in size in order to facilitate the passage through the birth canal.

Both the baby and mother can be left in a state of shock after a short intense labour. The baby's head is usually a good shape with minimal moulding, but the effects of the rapid intense compression can be felt as a quality change (a feeling of shock and irritation) in the delicate and sensitive meninges surrounding the brain. Osteopaths call this 'traumatic membranous inertia'. These babies are generally extremely restless, fractious, do not like to be put down, and cry a great deal.

This effect can occasionally be present in a baby that has had a very long labour. Normally the baby's head descends deep into the pelvis, (engages) before the onset of labour. However, occasionally the head may not engage until very late even though the labour may have gone on for some time. The baby may then experience sudden head compression without sufficient time for moulding to occur gently, and can suffer the same type of stresses as in a very rapid labour.

Strength of contractions

In a long labour, contractions can be both weak and ineffective, or strong. They may be strong but rather unco-ordinated, so that they act inefficiently on the cervix (or neck) of the uterus and it dilates slowly. In a rapid labour the contractions are usually very strong and well co-ordinated, working efficiently to open up the cervix. As a result the baby's head has to mould in a shorter length of time.

Induced labours are often accompanied by very strong contractions, and because the cervix may not be ready to dilate, the labour continues very strongly against resistance. This increases compressive forces on the baby's head. A slower steady labour is generally better for the baby.

Size of the baby's head

In general the size of the baby's head does not make a great deal of difference to the compressive forces on it, unless the head is very large. Small babies can be as difficult to deliver as large ones! The size of the mother's pelvis is important in determining how large a baby she can deliver with ease. Unless a mother has a large pelvis, a large baby (over 9-10lbs) can suffer more moulding than a small baby as it is necessary for the head to reduce relatively more in size to be able to pass through the pelvis.

The size of the birth canal is usually directly related to limitations within the mother's pelvis, such as those already described. Scar tissue from a previous labour can limit the size of the birth canal, but this is usually offset by the fact that the birth canal offers much less resistance to expansion in second or subsequent deliveries.

Pain relieving drugs

Labour is often described as the most painful experience in life. Most mothers need some form of pain relief in order to be able to cope. Some of these affect the baby as well and the effects of some, like Pethidine, can have a lasting effect on the baby. This does not mean that mothers should feel obliged not to have pain relief if they need it, or guilty if they have had it – the effects are treatable in the baby. However, it is important for the osteopath to know what pain relief the mother had during labour, to assist them in understanding the physical state of the baby.

Gas and air

This has no known effect on the baby during labour.

Pethidine

Pethidine is often given to the mother in labour, the effects last for up to approximately four hours in the mother. It also passes into the baby's blood stream, and both mother and baby experience the effect of the drug. Pethidine not only reduces pain, it also makes both mother and baby very sleepy. If the Pethidine is given to the mother near to delivery, the baby may still be in a drugged and sleepy state when it is born. This may mean that the baby does not take a really good first breath at birth to open up the lungs. This can interfere with the establishment of a good breathing pattern and prevent the baby from learning to use the lungs to their full capacity. Many osteopaths feel that this contributes to chest problems such as asthma later in life.

A newborn baby's liver is relatively immature, and does not cope with eliminating the effects of Pethidine as well as in an adult. Thus the effects of Pethidine may last much longer in a newborn baby than in his/her mother. It may make the baby particularly sleepy for up to a week and the effects may be present in the body for much longer.

If a baby is unduly sleepy in the first few days of life, breastfeeding is more difficult to get established, and bonding with the mother may delayed or interfered with. In addition the normal unmoulding process after birth is compromised. Crying, yawning and suckling assist the unmoulding process, and sleepy babies do not do much of the crying or suckling!

Osteopathic treatment can assist the unmoulding process in the head after birth, and treatment to release tension in the rib cage and diaphragm can improve lung function.

Epidural
An epidural is a local anaesthetic that is injected around the spinal cord of the mother, to numb the nerves to the uterus. Commonly the legs are numbed as well, so mothers who have had an epidural are generally confined to bed for the duration of labour. The anaesthetic is absorbed only slowly into the mother's blood stream, and the baby gets little of the effect of the drug. The baby may be rather jumpy for a few days after birth after an epidural, but there is no known lasting effect.

The labour of a mother who has an epidural carries an increased chance of needing forceps or ventouse to assist delivery of the baby for a variety of reasons; the muscles of the pelvic floor are relaxed by the anaesthetic, which makes them inefficient at guiding the baby's head through some of the rotation necessary for its descent through the pelvis.

With an epidural the mother cannot move around freely in labour. Long periods of time spent in the common reclining position limit the normal 'opening up' of the pelvis during the first stage of labour. Changes of position of the mother during second stage can be helpful in assisting the head to descend and rotate through the pelvis, and this is generally not possible with an epidural.

The mother may not be able to feel an urge to push in second stage and thus may not be able to synchronise her pushes with the uterine contractions. This causes greater pressure on the baby, and is less effective in pushing it down the birth canal.

It is common for a mother to suffer from ongoing back problems after having an epidural in labour. Normally we move in response to discomfort in the back, which is a self-protection mechanism. With an epidural the mother has no sensation of pain from the waist down, so is unaware of normal back discomfort. She may be in one position for many hours with intensely strong contractions exerting large forces on her pelvis from the inside. This can cause strain of some of the pelvic ligaments and a displacement of the normal position of the sacrum within the pelvis afterwards. Osteopathic treatment may be necessary to correct this.

The position of the baby's head
The position of the baby's head in relation to the mother's pelvis is called the presentation.

Normal presentation
The baby normally presents head downwards and facing backwards towards the mother's spine, with his/her chin tucked well down onto the chest. This offers the smallest diameter of the head to the birth canal, and gives the best chance of the baby passing smoothly through the birth canal.

Unusual or abnormal presentations
Sometimes the head is incompletely tucked down, or presents at a slightly odd angle. This not only slows the labour, but also presents a larger diameter of the head to the birth canal. This results in greater compressive forces being applied to parts of the head that are not well designed to take it.

To demonstrate the difference, it may help to imagine that you are pulling on a tight polo neck jumper, and consider the difference between having your head tipped backwards pulling it over your face first, or having your chin tucked down and pulling it over the top of your head. The smallest diameter is with the chin well tucked down onto the chest, the largest from chin to the crown of the head.

Posterior presentation
A common presentation is for the baby to present in a posterior position. In this position the mother and baby have their spines in contact with each other, with the baby facing forwards. They are literally lying back to back.

From the baby's point of view delivery from a posterior position is more difficult than from the normal anterior position. The head has to turn through three-quarters of a turn within the confines of the pelvis, to be delivered easily. The baby often gets stuck at this stage, and needs assistance. The baby's head is subjected to very complex forces in this type of delivery, and inevitably these are absorbed in addition to the normal compressive forces.

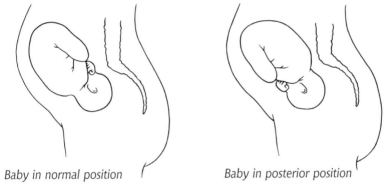

Baby in normal position   Baby in posterior position

Face presentation

The most difficult presentation for both mother and baby is a face presentation. The neck is fully extended or tipped back, and the maximum possible diameter of the head is presented. Moulding is extreme, and severe retained compression is inevitable.

Breech position

Babies are not designed to come out bottom first. In a breech presentation the head does not get a chance to mould during labour, and is delivered with the forces directed upwards instead of downwards. There are particular patterns of retained compression found in breech babies.

In a breech delivery, the baby's pelvis is subjected to large compressive forces as it is pushed into the cervix of the uterus, which it is not designed to take. This can leave retained distortion and compression in the sacrum and pelvis, which remains as the child grows and can alter the shape of the developing pelvis.

Following a breech delivery the baby may have difficulty learning to sit because the shape of the pelvis is altered by the compressive forces applied to it. Later on there may be a vulnerability to back problems. In a girl, it may even influence the shape of the pelvis enough to make delivery of her own children difficult.

An osteopath can readily treat the effects on the whole body of breech delivery.

First baby

Generally first babies have the hardest time in forcing a way through the mother's pelvis. The cervix of the uterus has not opened up before, the birth canal has not been stretched, nor the joints of the pelvis separated. For these reasons, first labours are usually longer with stronger contractions, and usually carry a greater need for analgesic drugs.

This is reflected in the greater incidence and severity of retained moulding found in first children, assuming the labours have been normal. It is an interesting observation that first children are commonly the most fractious and difficult babies in families! Some of this at least is due to the greater amount of birth compression they usually experience.

Assisted deliveries – forceps or ventouse

If the baby gets stuck at any stage in the delivery, or sometimes because they are in a state of distress, the delivery may need to be assisted with either forceps or ventouse (suction) appliances.

When these appliances are used, the baby is already stuck or in distress, and the head is under maximum compression. This means that maximum natural moulding has already occurred, and the extra compression inevitably applied to the head can be very difficult for the baby to release afterwards.

Forceps and ventouse deliveries are at times life saving, but they invariably cause increased compression on the baby's head, which rarely releases unaided after birth.

Babies that are born prematurely or overdue

The baby's head is best designed to withstand the compressive forces of birth at 40 weeks gestation.

Overdue babies

After 40 weeks of pregnancy the bones of the baby's head gradually harden so that they are not able to change shape or mould as easily during labour. This means that more of the compression is taken up within and between the bones, and is more difficult for the baby to release afterwards unaided.

Prematurity

In babies who are born before 37 weeks of pregnancy, the bones are very soft and suffer more from the compressive forces of labour, in spite of the small size of the head.

After birth the baby's head is subjected to the forces of gravity when the bones are still very soft, and not yet designed to cope with it. They often develop flattened sides of their heads as a result of this. Premature babies have many problems to overcome as a result of their early entry into the world, one of which is the effect of moulding pressures of labour and life outside the uterus before they are ready for it. Some of the effects of this are discussed in the next chapter.

Foetal distress

Babies occasionally suffer a shortage of oxygen during labour. This is known as 'foetal distress'. Mothers are carefully monitored during labour to detect signs of distress before it is severe enough to cause any lasting problem to the baby. However, sometimes they do suffer a significant amount of distress. The effect can vary in degree from minor distress causing hypoxia (minor shortage of oxygen), to serious anoxia that can lead to brain damage.

There are a variety of effects that hypoxia or anoxia can have on a baby and developing child. In the most mild cases there may be no sign of it at all, or there may be perhaps a learning difficulty of some sort, perhaps a difficulty in co-ordination, or an undermining of general health leading to fatigue and increased vulnerability to infection. More severe effects of anoxia may be cerebral palsy, in all its degrees from mild to severe.

Anoxia is always accompanied by a degree of shock to the central nervous system (brain) of the baby. This is a major factor in limiting the release of the moulding pressures after birth. It is also true that if the labour has been difficult enough to cause anoxia, it has usually also been physically hard on the baby, with a lot of moulding and compressive forces.

Children who suffer from cerebral palsy as a result of anoxia during their birth often have very small and odd shaped heads. This is partly because brain damage slows growth and development of the brain, so that the container (the skull) also grows more slowly. It is also because there may be a lot of retained moulding from a long and traumatic birth.

Much can be done to help these children with osteopathic treatment, to release the retained moulding and compression, as well as reducing (as far as possible) the effect on the nervous system. This is discussed in greater depth in the next chapter.

Cord round the neck

The umbilical cord frequently becomes wrapped around the baby during pregnancy, as the baby moves around. It is fairly common for it to become wrapped around the neck. This means that during delivery, the cord can tighten and restrict descent of the baby's head through the pelvis. Usually this causes no problem as the cord is generally loose enough to be hooked over the baby's head after the head is delivered and before the body, Occasionally it is so tightly wrapped around the neck that it has to be cut before the baby can be delivered.

The effects of the cord around the neck are varied:

• It may reduce or cut off the supply of blood to the baby, and cause the heart rate to drop to a greater or lesser extent. This may be severe enough to cause some anoxic effects.

• The strangulation effect of the cord can set up reflex irritation in the throat, which can make the throat very oversensitive.

These children may be very fearful and often hate having their neck touched. They are occasionally so distressed that they constantly throw their head back or claw at their neck with their hands. As they grow up, they are often very fussy about lumpy food and may like their food pureed well beyond the normal six months. They usually hate wearing anything tight around their neck.

Caesarean birth

After reading all the above, it may seem that every baby should be born by caesarean section! In some cases it is a preferable type of delivery if the delivery is likely to be very difficult. However, the baby does benefit from the normal birth process. It is a very stimulating time for them. It is a form of 'awakening' for the baby.

In many of the babies that we see who have had a caesarean birth there is still retained compression in their heads. This is particularly true if the caesarean is performed after a long period of labour. In addition the actual delivery by caesarean may not be easy especially if the baby's head is wedged deep in the pelvis.

Part of the moulding process and compression of the infant head begins in late pregnancy, so even the babies born by planned caesarean with no labour at all may have areas of compression.

Babies born by a planned caesarean where they have not been in labour at all are often very sleepy in the first few days. They may be unresponsive and seemingly in a world of their own, as they have not been 'woken up' by labour. Later on they may display a degree of shock from being born unprepared, and this often makes them clingy children who may be reluctant to approach new situations.

After caesarean delivery milk production in the mother is usually slower to establish. This may make it more difficult to establish breastfeeding, especially if the baby is unduly sleepy in the first few days.

Emotional effects of labour on the baby

Babies are aware of the atmosphere around the birth. If it is calm and serene, and the mother is coping well, the baby may have a peaceful and joyful arrival into the world. If there is anxiety, stress or panic, the baby may detect this and hold on to a level of anxiety afterwards. This is often released during osteopathic treatment with effective release of the physical strains associated with birth.

Babies that have had a difficult passage during labour, particularly if they have been stuck at any point, often become very frightened. This is quite different from the foetal distress caused by a shortage of oxygen in labour. It can affect them later on, often manifesting in a physical state as tension through the diaphragm and chest, and in an emotional way by making them tense, nervy individuals. Such babies and children may be clingy and fearful, particularly of new situations, and often need a lot of reassurance from their parents and carers.

5

Effects of retained moulding on the baby

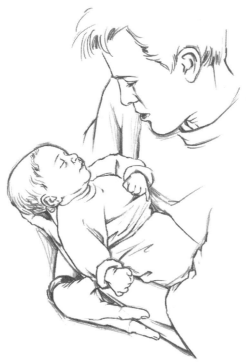

*W*e have looked at the kind of things in pregnancy and labour that can lead to retained moulding in a baby or child. It is now time to move on and look at what this means from the baby's point of view.

Everyone has his or her own opinion as to what is wrong with a baby when he/she is crying. It can be very difficult for new parents, especially the mother and particularly if it is her first child, to try to make sense of the enormous amount of conflicting advice that inevitably comes her way.

A new mother may feel a sense of inadequacy or even a feeling of failure as a mother if her baby cries incessantly, will not sleep, or feeding is difficult. It may seem that everyone else's baby sleeps through the night, and is relaxed and contented except hers.

These mothers may at the same time have a sense of unease about their child, or be worried that something is really wrong with the child but that no one will listen to her. It can be a very lonely and isolating time. It is not surprising that some of these mothers get depressed.

Many parents are delighted when they visit an osteopath to find out that something really is wrong with their baby, and that it is easily treatable (usually!). Most people who have had children of their own will read the following section and either recognise some of the signs of retained moulding in their own children, or know of several babies or children who have these signs. They are extremely common.

Crying, irritable baby

All babies cry to some extent, but some more than others. Babies that cry a lot, or have a particularly piercing cry may be suffering from retained birth compression. The baby's head may be uncomfortable, possibly with a headache.

Uncomfortable babies may not only cry a lot, be restless and fractious, they may also be jumpy especially with loud noises, and take a long time to settle to sleep. They are typically more comfortable being carried than lying down, because the extra pressure of the mattress on their head aggravates the pressure already in their head. This will probably then wake them up. They are not simply being naughty and wanting lots of cuddles. However, the need to be cuddled to sleep will become habit forming if it persists. Babies who have had a very rapid labour are often the most fractious, irritable babies.

Babies who have been stuck in the birth canal or who have had the cord wrapped around their neck are often very fearful babies, in constant need of reassurance. They prefer to be carried most of the time, and need to know that their mother is near.

Feeding

Many babies feed quickly and easily either from the breast or bottle, with a gap of three to four hours in between. Unfortunately this is not always the case. Some babies are very slow feeders and one feed may merge into the next. The baby may fall asleep before he/she has taken a full feed, and therefore wakes hungry after an hour or two.

The baby may be a 'windy' feeder. A 'snack and nap' habit can develop which is not good for digestion, for maintaining a good supply of milk if breastfeeding, or for getting periods of deep and restful sleep (for both parents and baby).

Parents may also notice that the baby feeds more easily on one side than the other. This may be a sign that he/she has some residual strain in the neck from labour and delivery, and can turn more easily to one side than the other.

A baby that fusses and fidgets when feeding may be displaying signs of discomfort in the back of the head and top of the neck. Care should be taken not to inadvertently make this worse by resting the baby's head on anything hard during feeding, such as a bony forearm.

The nerve to the tongue that controls the suckling action exits from the skull in an area behind the ear. This is the area that takes the maximum compression during the passage down the birth canal. The nerve may be irritated and this can affect the function of the tongue muscles making suckling difficult and tiring. These babies may be described as having a 'weak suck'. They may also be having difficulty co-ordinating the action of sucking with swallowing.

Other factors that can make suckling difficult are:
- moulding of the whole skull leaving residual stress through the face.
- irritation in the throat caused by the umbilical cord being tightly wrapped around the neck.
- stress and discomfort in the throat if it has been over-stretched by the head being tipped backwards during delivery, such as caused by a face or brow presentation.

A baby that is finding feeding difficult may be slow to gain weight.

Getting breastfeeding established

Getting breastfeeding established in the early days and weeks can be difficult, but the enormous advantages for the baby of breastfeeding over bottle-feeding make it worth the effort. The nutritional advantages of breast milk over bottle are well known. Less well understood is the fact that the action of breastfeeding is a lot more helpful to the baby in releasing the effects of birth compression that the easier action of bottle feeding.

Many mother and baby partnerships do not manage to overcome the initial problems of breastfeeding. In some cases, it may appear that the mother does not have enough milk to satisfy the baby, but it may be that the problem arises from the baby's difficulty in suckling correctly. This in turn may be the result of retained birth compression in the baby, making it difficult for him/her to latch on and suckle correctly.

If the baby is not latched on correctly, this may cause sore and cracked nipples because the baby 'chews' on the nipple rather than sucking with the nipple well back in his/her mouth. In addition, the incorrect sucking action will not stimulate the mother's milk production. The baby may tire before he has taken a full feed, sleep for a short time and then wake up hungry again. Or the baby may still seem hungry after feeds so the occasional top-up bottle may then be introduced, which the baby seems to prefer because he/she does not have to work so hard for the milk. Gradually a pattern is established of the baby spending less time at the breast, and the lack of stimulation reduces breast milk production so that the supply dwindles further. Eventually the baby may reject the breast totally in favour of the bottle.

Babies who early on reject the breast in favour of the bottle may do so because they have such a degree of retained compression that breastfeeding is difficult, and the easier option of bottle-feeding is less tiring.

Osteopathic treatment as soon as possible after birth may be a great help in getting breastfeeding established.

Self-help breast-feeding tips

The first two points may also be relevant for a bottle-fed baby.
- If your baby appears to fight the breast, ie gets very agitated shortly after he/she has latched on, this may be because of discomfort in the feeding position. It may be difficult for him to turn towards the breast

on one side. Try to notice whether this occurs more when he is feeding from one side than the other. If so, try tucking his feet under your arm in a rugby ball type of position so that his head is turning to his easy side.

• The back of the head and neck can be very sensitive in babies. Be careful not to put pressure on the back of his/her head or neck with your arm.

• It can be difficult to know whether a baby that seems to want to feed for very long periods is really feeding or just comfort sucking. One way to tell is to count the number of times that they swallow. If they suck and suck but rarely swallow, it is probably comfort sucking. This is fine in moderation, but you may prefer to use a dummy or allow them to suck on your (clean) finger instead of the breast.

• Try to make your baby go at least 2 hours between feeds, otherwise the whole pattern becomes very disrupted and you are never quite sure what is a feed and what is a snack.

Infantile colic

Most people instantly diagnose a crying baby as having colic, or teething. In reality colic is only one of the reasons a baby may cry incessantly, as has already been discussed. However, colic is a very painful reality for some babies. Studies have shown that 25-40% of babies suffer from colic, which can vary from mild to severe. Severe colic may account for up to 15% of these babies.[4,5,6.] Both breast and bottle fed babies can suffer from colic.

Colic is often referred to as 'three month colic', indicating that it resolves by three months of age. There certainly is a natural improvement over time, but many babies continue to suffer colic well past three months of age. A survey in 1982[7] showed that only 47% of babies with colic had improved by 3 months, another 41% had improved by 6 months, but 12% of babies with colic still had symptoms of colic at 1 year.

Some facts about colic:

Evening crying

Colic is often referred to as 'evening colic'. Research has shown that only 20% of babies with colic show the evening crying pattern, that is commonly associated with it.[7]

Mother's diet
In a breast-fed infant, foods in the mother's diet may cause or aggravate colic. Foods such as brassicas, bananas and acid fruit, wheat and spicy food are best avoided. Research has shown that a low allergen diet in the mother can help a colicky infant.[8]

Lactose intolerance
Some babies have a lactose intolerance, which causes colic.[9] Lactose is present in cows milk and dairy products, and if this is suspected to be a cause of colic in a breast-fed baby, the mother should avoid dairy products in her diet. In bottle fed babies soya milk formula may relieve the colic. Special preparations of hydrolysed casein can help those babies with severe milk intolerance. This is normally available on prescription.

Stress in pregnancy
Research has shown a significant association between stress in pregnancy and colic in the infant.[2]

Siblings
Babies with colic are more likely to have siblings who have also suffered from colic.[2]

Osteopathic treatment is effective for colic
Osteopaths feel that mechanical stresses imposed on the baby during pregnancy and delivery can cause or aggravate colic. In 1996 Clive Hayden DO performed a controlled clinical trial on the efficacy of osteopathic treatment for infantile colic.[10] The trial showed that osteopathy is highly effective at reducing the symptoms of infantile colic. Babies who had received treatment slept longer and cried less than those who did not.

There are a number of reasons why osteopathy can help colic. There is no single technique that is effective, and an osteopath treats all areas where dysfunction is found.

A common area where dysfunction is found in babies with colic is in the base of the skull behind the ear. The nerve to the stomach exits from the skull in this region, and this area is particularly vulnerable to compression during a normal birth. Retained compression here can irritate the nerve, impair the efficiency of digestion and interfere with normal digestion in the stomach.

The diaphragm can be affected by stress through the trunk of the baby from its passage through the birth canal, from shock from the birth, or a poor first breath. Any impairment in the function of the diaphragm has a major effect on the ability of the stomach to retain and digest its contents. If the umbilical cord has been subjected to tension during delivery, perhaps because it was wrapped around the baby's neck, this can disturb the function of the diaphragm. Problems in this area will manifest frequently as windy or colicky babies.

A baby who has been subjected to stress in pregnancy via his/her mother will have a more reactive nervous system, and this is thought to contribute to the increased vulnerability to colic in these infants. Osteopathic treatment is effective at generally relaxing the baby, which reduces the reactivity of the whole nervous system including the nerve supply of the stomach and intestines. This often reduces colicky symptoms of discomfort and crying.

Sickness in babies

The stomach is held shut at its upper end by a muscular ring or 'sphincter' formed by muscle fibres from the diaphragm. Stress or distortion in the diaphragm can impede the efficiency of this sphincter and cause the baby to bring back small amounts of milk when the stomach is full after feeds. Osteopathic treatment to balance the tension around the diaphragm often reduces the amount of regurgitation of milk.

A sphincter called the pyloric sphincter closes the lower end of the stomach. Rarely this sphincter is structurally deficient, and remains tightly closed. This is called pyloric stenosis. In this condition whole feeds are repeatedly regurgitated, because the milk cannot escape from the lower end of the stomach. This has to be corrected by surgery.

Thumb sucking and dummies

Sucking is one way that the baby can help to reduce his or her own moulding in the early days. This is one reason for the comfort sucking of a young baby. If this fails to achieve the desired release, the child may come to use thumb sucking or a dummy as a way of relieving the effects of the residual tension in his/her head. Ultimately this sucking is pure habit. This has long term implications on dental development as it alters the shape of the growing face.

Some breastfed babies seem to spend very long periods of time feeding which is time consuming, and can cause sore nipples and colic due to overfeeding. Often the baby is not feeding but simply comfort sucking, or

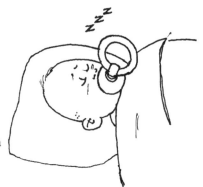

trying to release birth compression.
One way to tell if this is the case is to
count the number of times the baby
swallows. If he is sucking but rarely
swallowing, the feeding is probably
more for comfort. For these babies,
sucking on a clean finger or a dummy
may be better than using the breast as a
dummy. There is usually a natural time
to wean a baby off a dummy at around
8-12 weeks old, and using a dummy
early on certainly does not mean that a child will be dummy dependent
for years.

After 3 months or so, it becomes much more difficult to wean the baby
off the dummy because its use becomes habitual.

In the long term dentists generally find that there is less damage to
dental development from using a dummy than thumb sucking, because
thumb sucking generally places leverage on the teeth and pulls the dental
arch out of shape. Some 'orthodontic' dummies claim to reduce the
detrimental effects of sucking on the developing teeth.

Ideally children should have osteopathic treatment as young as possible
to relieve moulding compression, before sucking becomes purely a habit.
Although the moulding effects can be treated later, a habit can be very
hard to break.

Sleep disturbances

The close link of between sleeping and feeding patterns of the young baby
has already been discussed. A baby who does not take adequate milk at
one feed will need to wake sooner for the next feed. This can easily
develop into a 'snacking and napping' habit.

There are other things that can interfere with the sleeping patterns of
babies. Discomfort in the head may prevent the baby falling into a really
deep sleep, so shutting out everything in the outside world. In addition the
stresses of retained compression on the bony casing of the skull may be
transmitted via the coverings of the brain (the meninges) to the brain itself.
As a result the baby's nervous system may be kept in a persistently alert
state. These babies sleep for only short periods at a time, and never seem
to fall into a deep sleep. Later in the first year they are awakened by the
slightest noise.

These sleeping patterns gradually become habit forming. If the baby is treated to release the retained birth compression when young, then this alone may be sufficient to solve the sleeping problem.

After the first year, even after the causative problem of the birth compression has been treated, this habit pattern may need working on separately by the parents. This may involve a few nights of being firm with the baby, just popping in and out to reassure him/her of the parent's presence but not picking him/her up.

Sleep patterns may be disturbed by teething, infections, and as a result of accidents. The effects of falls such as bangs to the head can disturb the body mechanics in a similar way to the trauma of birth, and cause discomfort in the head, or simply stresses that keep the nervous system in an aroused state which prevents the child sleeping soundly. It is common for a child to succumb to an infection after a traumatic fall, because the immune system is temporarily disarmed by the shock of the fall. Osteopathic treatment can be effective at releasing the physical effects of teething or accidents, and allows the child to settle back into a normal sleep pattern.

Head scratching and banging

Young babies sometimes claw at their head with their hands and scratch themselves, often in one particular part of the head. This may be caused by skin irritation such as eczema, but is often an indication that the head is uncomfortable from retained birth moulding.

Head banging in a baby or young child can simply be caused by frustration or temper. However in many of these children, they are suffering from the effects of retained compression from birth. The head banging is an attempt by the child to relieve some of the pressure and discomfort in the head. Head banging usually stops after treatment of the underlying compression.

Head shape

The wide variety of head shapes amongst babies is very obvious to the trained eye, and often to the untrained eye. Parents may be understandably very concerned about significant asymmetry. Asymmetry of head shape is the result of moulding either in pregnancy or during birth and can have far reaching consequences. It is commonly accompanied by spinal asymmetry and scoliosis, and can contribute to long term spinal problems. It is also associated with abnormal dental occlusion patterns. All babies with asymmetrical heads should be checked by an osteopath as early as possible.

Occasionally the head is a good shape after birth, but as the child grows a marked asymmetry develops. In this case it is because areas of retained compression from pregnancy or birth have affected the way the bone can grow. Bone growth is greatest in areas where there is no strain within the bone, and least where in areas of retained stress within the bone.

Osteopathic treatment may produce quite dramatic changes to head symmetry if it is carried out soon after birth when the bones are still very supple. When the child is a little older, the shape usually persists even after the moulding stresses are released, although asymmetry may reduce a little as the bone continues to grow unimpeded.

The most difficult head shape to correct is that caused by moulding during pregnancy, where the head has been pressed against some bony part of the mother over a long period of time. The bone moulds to the shape of the structures around it. During osteopathic treatment there may be minimal stress palpable in the bone structure, and it can be difficult to change.

Head asymmetry in itself is not a problem if it is well compensated within the body. Osteopaths are far more concerned about balance and harmony in all body tissues than about symmetry. If head asymmetry is well compensated by all structures in the body, then it is of no long-term significance. Osteopaths often find more problems in an apparently symmetrical and well-shaped head.

Eventually of course a baby grows hair which hides much of the asymmetry, but it does not disappear – just look around you at some adult faces and you will see many interesting examples.

Emotional link of the baby with the mother

A young baby is very emotionally linked with his/her mother. Many mothers have noticed that if they are feeling tired or down, the baby will have a fractious day. If the mother is suffering ongoing emotional stress herself, perhaps in a relationship, bereavement, anxiety or stress of any sort, the baby may pick up on this. In these cases even after the retained moulding compression is released, the baby may still be unsettled.

It may be necessary for the mother to have treatment herself, either osteopathic or other appropriate treatment, in order to help the baby relax.

Teething

Some babies seem to cut teeth with no problem. For others teething causes great suffering with a variety of symptoms such as teething pain and discomfort, disrupted sleep, colds and chest infections, or skin problems such as eczema or nappy rash, over many days and weeks.

The eruption of teeth involves relatively rapid movement of teeth within the bones of the face. This often causes a degree of strain and tension within the face bones, the effects of which can be transmitted to other parts of the head. Any tension already present from retained birth moulding is likely to be aggravated. Therefore a baby who has had a difficult birth is more likely to suffer badly with teething. Osteopathic treatment can relieve both the tension caused by teething, and also the retained birth moulding. This usually dramatically reduces the disruption to the health and well being of the baby with teething.

Effects of prematurity

Modern technology is enabling babies to survive from a much younger age than has been possible in the past. These babies have specific difficulties not experienced by full term infants.

The main problem experienced by premature babies is with breathing. Their lungs are immature and not ready to function. If premature delivery is inevitable the mother is often given steroids for a few days before birth, which helps to reduce these breathing difficulties. In spite of this, all very young babies (born before 30 weeks) and some of the more mature (30-35 weeks) need help from a ventilator to breathe.

The stress on the lungs of being inflated and used so young can scar the lungs and leave a lasting weakness. They often remain small, and feel hard and inelastic on osteopathic palpation. This may make the child vulnerable to chest infections and asthma. Another consideration is the ventilator itself. If it has been used for some time, there may be a degree of moulding in the face and head around the ventilator tube itself. This may create stress through the face that needs releasing later.

Babies born before 35-36 weeks do not have a sucking reflex, and as it develops they find it difficult to co-ordinate the action of sucking and swallowing. Very premature babies are fed directly into the blood stream. Less vulnerable babies are tube fed straight into the stomach to start with, and have to learn to suckle later on. They are often very slow feeders, and may never develop a strong sucking action. This may be improved by treatment to release any compression in the base of the skull, and through

63

the face.

The moulding of the heads of premature babies has already been discussed. This moulding and compression in the head can contribute to such things as developmental delay and learning difficulties, hyperactivity, recurrent ear infections, and overcrowding of teeth. These are discussed in Chapter 8.

Babies who are born very prematurely suffer very high levels of shock and stress as a result of being forcibly thrust into the world and having to struggle for survival, at a time when they should be protected and secure within the uterus. They are deprived of the reassuring presence of their mother, and their environment is one of wires, tubes and machines. This stress is palpable osteopathically often into adulthood, and can render these individuals less able to cope with further stress in life.

Osteopathic treatment can be of great benefit in helping these babies both during their early and most vulnerable time, and as they grow later on. Great care and skill is needed when treating sick, premature babies, as they are very over sensitive to any interference. However, very short treatments and the most gentle of approaches can be beneficial in helping to reduce shock in their system, which then helps them to become less hypersensitive. A sick premature baby is wired up to machines that monitor heart rate, blood gasses, respiration etc. Nurses often comment how these readings improve after osteopathic treatment. As the baby becomes less unstable, treatments can be increased accordingly.

6

Postnatal care of the mother

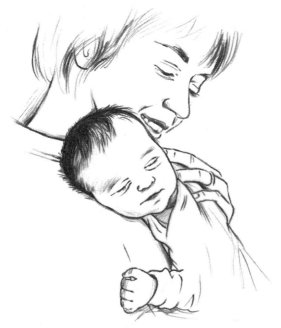

*W*ith the excitement and exhaustion of the first few days and weeks with a new baby, parents are usually focussed wholly on meeting the baby's needs. It is easy to forget that the mother's body is going through some major changes as it recovers from both the pregnancy and the birth.

The care and nurturing of a young family is an unrelenting 24 hour a day, 365 days a year job. The demands continue no matter how the mother is feeling, so she has a responsibility to take good care of her own health in order to be able to meet these demands. Osteopathy has a very important place in helping a new mother to recover physically and mentally from the pregnancy and labour.

Physical recovery from pregnancy and childbirth is not always straightforward, and is often incomplete if the physical demands of the pregnancy have been great, or the birth difficult. This can lead to a wide variety of problems both in the short term and in the long term, many of which can be prevented with appropriate osteopathic treatment.

This chapter looks at the common problems that osteopaths encounter in mothers after childbirth, and how treatment can help.

The demands of labour on the mother's body

Labour is an extremely physically demanding activity, and although it is a natural process it can place the mother's body under great strain.

The baby's head is a tight fit in the maternal pelvis, and as the baby descends and passes through the birth canal, the mother's pelvis is vulnerable to being distorted and its ligaments overstrained. This can cause difficulties during labour, in the immediate postnatal period, or in the long term.

Pelvic strain during childbirth

The pelvis is designed to adapt during labour to allow more space for the passage of the baby's head. To achieve this, the bones of the pelvis spread apart slightly, the sacrum moves backwards away from the baby's head, and the coccyx hinges backwards from its normal position at the tip of the sacrum. In addition the softening of the ligaments in the mother's body during pregnancy allows the bones of the pelvis to separate slightly during delivery. These mechanisms can increase the size of the 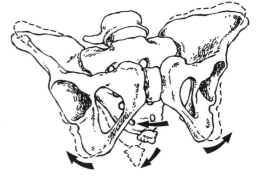 pelvic outlet by as much as 30%, but even with this the passage of the head is a tight fit as it passes through the mother's pelvis during a normal vaginal delivery.

The passage of the baby's head can force any part of the pelvis out of its normal position, leaving the pelvic bones strained and unbalanced, or the sacrum or coccyx stuck in an unnatural position. This can set up a variety of problems in the future, which will be discussed later in the chapter.

Situations that predispose to pelvic strain during childbirth

Pre-existing strains within the pelvis that limit its ability to spread to allow the passage of the baby

The importance of osteopathic treatment during pregnancy to balance and reduce pre-existing strains within the pelvis has already been discussed in chapter 2. If these strains and stresses are not treated before labour begins, they can limit the ability of the parts of the pelvis to separate and move out of the way in labour. This may make the labour more difficult for both mother and baby, and it also increases the likelihood of overstrain of all or part of the pelvis during labour. Osteopathic treatment in pregnancy aims to ensure that the pelvis is ready and able to adapt to the demands of labour by reducing excessive muscular tension, resolving any ligamentous imbalance, and finding the optimum structural balance of the pelvis.

Position of the mother in labour

Ideally the mother should find her most comfortable position in labour, because that is usually the one that places least strain on her own body. Generally mothers prefer upright or leaning forward positions because these relieve pressure on the sacrum. These positions also facilitate the normal separation and expansion of the pelvis, thus making delivery of the baby easier.

Normally the sacrum swings backwards at its lower end to increase the size of the pelvic outlet and move the coccyx out of the way of the baby's head. This adaptive movement is restricted if the mother spends much of the labour in a reclining position where her weight is taken on the sacrum most of the time. As a result the passage of the baby's head as it is driven into the curve of the sacrum may drag the sacrum out of its normal position.

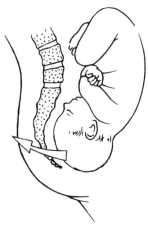

If the abnormal position of the sacrum is not corrected in the first few weeks after labour, then as the mother's ligaments return to normal after the pregnancy the sacrum can become fixed in this malposition. This can have a number of consequences, both immediately and in the long term, which will be discussed later in this chapter.

A large baby, or a small or misshapen pelvis
Occasionally a mother's pelvis is misshapen so that it is impossible for a baby to pass through. This is called pelvic disproportion, and a caesarean delivery is a necessity. More commonly the bony pelvic shape is not ideal but distortion is not extreme, and the mother may be offered a 'trial of labour', i.e. labour is allowed to begin normally but if no progress is made a caesarean is performed. In a first pregnancy pelvic disproportion may only be diagnosed after delivery, if the labour fails to progress. In this event the mother's pelvis may be x-rayed after delivery to establish whether pelvic disproportion is present, in which case a caesarean can be planned in any future pregnancy.

A very large baby in proportion to the size of the mother, or a baby with a large head may also make the delivery more difficult. In both cases, whilst osteopathy cannot remove the problem, osteopathic treatment during pregnancy to optimise pelvic function can offer the best chance of an uncomplicated delivery.

Epidural
An epidural is a local anaesthetic that is injected around the spinal cord that numbs the nerves to the uterus. Its effect is generally to numb everything from the waist down, although anaesthetists are becoming increasingly skilled at localising the area of numbness to the uterus alone.

The back is more vulnerable to injury during labour when the mother has an epidural. With an epidural, the mother normally rests in a semi-reclining position on the bed, sitting with pressure directly on her sacrum. She may be in this position for many hours and cannot feel discomfort in her back that would normally make her move. At the same time the uterus is contracting strongly and the baby descending through the pelvis, which adds pressure on the sacrum from the inside, with the result that the sacrum and its supporting ligaments can become strained or pulled out of position by the baby's head. If she were able to feel pain normally, the mother would naturally move to reduce this pressure, so reducing the likelihood of back strain.

If possible the epidural is allowed to wear off for the second stage of labour to help the mother push more effectively. If she is still numb from the epidural she cannot feel any urge to push, which makes it much harder for her to synchronise her pushing efforts with the contractions. This puts more strain on the mother's body and more pressure on the baby, and increases the likelihood of intervention such as forceps or ventouse being necessary to assist the delivery.

Occasionally a local irritation persists in the spinal meninges (coverings of the spinal cord) at site of epidural. This does not normally cause any undue problem, but mothers often state that they can feel the site of the epidural for some time afterwards. When combined with other physical strain from the pregnancy and birth, this irritation can contribute to back pain or headaches. Osteopathic treatment can help to reduce this irritation as well as correct the effect of physical strain and imbalance in the whole body after pregnancy and childbirth.

Lithotomy position (stirrups)

This inelegant position may be used for assisted deliveries such as forceps or ventouse deliveries, or for stitching the perineum after birth. It can add strain to the pelvic ligaments at a time that the pelvis is at its most vulnerable, either during delivery or immediately afterwards when it is floppy and unstable.

In traditional stirrups, it is only the ankles that are supported by straps and the weight of the legs tends to force the leg to drop outwards. This places a leverage on the two halves of the pelvis via the hips that can force the pelvic bones out of their correct alignment.

More modern stirrups are much improved and provide support for the whole calf, so preventing the legs dropping outwards. This greatly reduces the strain on the pelvis. Unfortunately they are not yet used in all hospitals.

Lithotomy strain is responsible for many cases of pelvic imbalance after childbirth, which can result on long-term back problems. It can also contribute to some gynaecological problems including painful or heavy periods; prolapse of the uterus where the uterus drops downwards onto the bladder because it is not well supported by its ligaments; or bladder problems including stress incontinence which is caused by disruption of pelvic floor muscles.

Pubic symphysis strain

The pubic symphysis is the name given to the ligamentous junction of the two halves of the pelvis in the front. As the baby's head is pushed through the pelvis and the two pelvic bones separated slightly during delivery, the ligaments of the pubic symphysis can be overstrained. In addition the two pelvic bones may be pulled out of position by the baby's head. If this is not corrected after delivery, the positional imbalance may persist and prevent full recovery of the overstrained ligaments of the pubic symphysis. This is called Diastasis Pubic Symphysis, and has already been discussed in chapter 2.

Osteopaths consider that pubic symphysis strain is more likely to occur when there is a restriction in the sacrum affecting the amount of 'give' in the sacroiliac ligaments on either side of the sacrum. These are the joints that can spread during labour, and if this spread is limited, the pubic symphysis ligaments may be forced to overstretch in compensation.

Osteopathic treatment is extremely effective at rebalancing the ligaments of the pelvis after labour and helping to resolve ongoing pubic symphysis pain after delivery.

Immediately after delivery

The separation of the pelvis during delivery of the baby leaves the pelvis very unstable immediately after delivery. In addition the pelvic floor muscles have been stretched to their limit, and sometimes beyond if the mother's perineum has torn or been cut during delivery.

Muscle pains (from stiff muscles) in any part of the body are common in the first few days after childbirth due to the physical effort involved in pushing the baby out. It can take enormous muscular effort from the mother to deliver the baby, and if she has not been pushing correctly down into the pelvic floor, this can involve any muscle of the body. These muscle pains normally resolve within a few days, but may persist if there is any postural imbalance as a result of the pregnancy or labour.

The strain of bearing down to push the baby out can leave tension locked in the rib cage. In particular, the shoulders may be left hunched forward and the rib cage held in a rounded shape as if tethered in the front at the bottom of the sternum (breastbone). This is due to residual tension in the diaphragm. It can cause a variety of symptoms – including breathing difficulties, postural strain with aching in the back, neck and shoulders, fatigue, headaches, heartburn, or aggravation of varicose veins or haemorrhoids because the return of blood back to the heart through the diaphragm is impaired. These stresses can be swiftly resolved with osteopathic treatment.

The abdominal muscles normally support the lumbar spine by forming a type of muscular corset around the whole abdomen. These muscles increase substantially in length during the pregnancy to accommodate the growing uterus. After delivery of the baby there is a sudden change in the mother's posture, and it takes several days for the muscles to shorten and regain their tone. This means that for the first few days the muscular support of the spine is poor, and the mother should take care not to overstrain her back such as by lifting the baby awkwardly, sitting in an asymmetrical position, or walking too far.

Feeding
In the early days much time is spent feeding the baby, and it is important for the mother to sit in a well-supported and comfortable position. When nursing a baby for a length of time it is easy to remain stuck in an awkward position, not wanting to move for fear of disturbing the baby. It is surprising how heavy even a very tiny baby can become after being held for a period of time. Sitting with the head bent forwards looking at the baby can cause back or neck ache. Any feeding position can be made more awkward if the mother finds sitting uncomfortable due to soreness from the delivery or from stitches.

Sitting in a well-supported position with the baby lying on a pillow to support his/her weight can help to reduce postural strain. It may take a little time to find a comfortable position for both mother and baby, especially when breastfeeding since the position of the baby is more critical than when bottle feeding. Some mothers find that it is easier to lie down and breastfeed, but even in this position care must be taken to support the

71

mother's neck, arms and spine.

Newborn babies are often sensitive to pressure on the back of the head and top of the neck, so in finding a good feeding position, care should be taken to support the baby's head on something soft, (not a bony arm). Be aware that if a baby fidgets or cries whilst feeding, it may be a sign of discomfort with the feeding position.

Mastitis is a common problem with breastfeeding. This arises initially due to a blocked milk duct that becomes inflamed and ultimately infected. This results in influenza like symptoms with the rapid development of fever, and a painful hot red area of the breast. Conventionally it is treated with antibiotics. Some women are vulnerable to repeated bouts of mastitis, that can be triggered either by getting overtired and run-down, by a poor feeding position so that one milk duct is not emptied during the feed, or by bruising such as from bumps by an over-enthusiastic toddler!

Osteopathic treatment can be effective in speeding up the recovery from mastitis, and if it is caught early enough, can reduce or eliminate the need for antibiotics. It can also help prevent recurrent bouts of mastitis. Treatment is aimed at improving lymphatic drainage from the breast and ensuring that the rib cage is freely mobile with no areas of restriction. This needs to be combined with changing the feeding position so that the baby fully drains the affected milk duct, and where necessary expressing milk from the affected duct after a feed to ensure that it is completely emptied.

The postnatal period

This period covers the first six weeks after delivery of the baby, which is the time when the body is returning to normal after the enormous demands of pregnancy and delivery.

Return of uterus to normal

In the first few days it is common for the mother to experience 'after-pains', which are due to the uterus contracting back to its normal size. The uterine contractions are stimulated by hormones released whist breastfeeding, so often occur during feeding. After-pains tend to get stronger with each pregnancy, and are likely to be worse if the uterus is twisted on its ligaments.

The uterus is suspended in its normal position in the pelvis by ligaments that attach to the walls of the pelvis and sacrum. These ligaments can become overstrained during pregnancy, by the forces of uterine contractions, or as a result of pelvic strain after childbirth. This can cause the uterus to return into an abnormal position as it reduces in size after childbirth – it can drop forwards, backwards or off to one side.

The pelvic floor muscles are also important in supporting the uterus and bladder in the correct position within the pelvis. The pelvic floor muscles are weakened during pregnancy, and overstretched by delivery. It is therefore vital to regain good pelvic floor muscle tone after childbirth, and pelvic floor exercises should be done frequently from the start.

Stress incontinence is so common as to be considered normal after childbirth. It is caused by a combination of:
- overstretch of the supporting ligaments of the bladder during labour
- additional pelvic strains from lithotomy position
- malposition of the uterus following childbirth
- weakened pelvic floor muscles

This distressing condition need not be inevitable after childbirth, provided the uterus and bladder are comfortably balanced within the pelvis, and pelvic floor muscles are exercised to regain good tone. Osteopathy can be invaluable in helping restore the position and balance of the uterus and bladder to normal after childbirth, and combined with exercises, this problem can usually be dramatically reduced or eliminated.

Uterine malposition can result in a wide variety of symptoms including prolonged or heavy bleeding after childbirth, painful or heavy periods, pain on intercourse, difficulty conceiving and a vulnerability to uterine or bladder prolapse in the future. Osteopathic treatment can help correct imbalance in the uterine ligaments and restore it to a more normal and comfortable position within the pelvis. In this way osteopathy can often help many of the above symptoms and prevent long-term problems in this area.

Postural changes after childbirth
After childbirth the body undergoes a rapid postural change to adapt to the dramatic reduction in size and weight of the uterus and contents. The posture should gradually return to normal in the first few weeks as muscles regain their normal tone, and ligaments shorten to their normal pre-pregnant length. If the position of the sacrum and pelvis has been disturbed during childbirth and is not corrected immediately, then as the ligaments return to their normal length they 'set' the pelvis in this abnormal position.

The pelvis and sacrum support the spine from the base, and any positional change here after childbirth disturbs the balance of the whole spine. The resultant change in the posture can still be seen many years later, and often leads to long-term back problems.

Flattened lumbar spine

During labour the sacrum may be pushed backwards at the upper end causing a marked change in the mother's normal posture thereafter. The pelvis remains stiff and the bottom tucked in, as if standing with an imaginary tail tucked between the legs. This flattens the curve in the lumbar (lower) spine and places strain on the lower back.

Hollow back

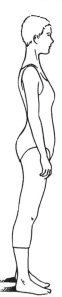

Alternatively the top of the sacrum can drop forwards and downwards into the pelvis during labour, giving a persistent hollow back and a protruding stomach. This posture is exaggerated if abdominal muscles are weak, because the spine lacks support from the front.

Long-term back pain

Malpositions of the sacrum and pelvis following childbirth not only cause postural changes, but can also restrict mobility in the lumbar spine. This can place undue load on the lumbar spine and if this situation persists it can lead to a range of back problems, anything from general backache to a more serious disc injury or early degeneration of the lumbar spine and premature arthritis.

Back pain may or may not arise immediately after childbirth, since the body is very good at accommodating areas of strain in the short term, and it is often only over a period of time that its ability to compensate is lost. It may be that a minor accident or fall some time later overloads the body's ability to cope, and problems arise. However, the origin can be traced back to postural change following childbirth.

Caesarean delivery

The body needs extra time to recover from a caesarean delivery. In addition to the normal healing from any abdominal surgery, the body is also recovering from pregnancy. The abdominal muscles have already been stretched and weakened by the pregnancy, and are then further weakened by the surgery. In addition the mother has to lift and care for her new baby, and even a newborn baby weighing 7lb can be difficult to lift without causing undue strain on the back in the first few days and weeks.

It is worth remembering that after similar abdominal surgery such as a hysterectomy, mothers are told not to drive or lift anything heavy for six weeks. Babies usually gain weight very rapidly, often gaining between 8oz and 1lb a week for the first few weeks. By six weeks old, they can be very heavy. If the baby is fractious and requires carrying around for long periods, this adds further load to the mother's weakened spine. Particular care should be taken when lifting the baby out of a cot, or a car seat in and out of the car.

Postnatal exercises after a caesarean delivery are extremely important for firstly shortening and then strengthening the abdominal muscles, in order to strengthen the spine. As soon as the scar is sufficiently healed, regular exercises should be undertaken, very gently at first, to build up the abdominal muscles.

Postnatal exercises and regaining fitness

First week:

There are many changes taking place in the mother's body in the first week after giving birth, and it is not necessary to do intensive postnatal exercises during this week.

- Pelvic floor muscles exercises should be done many times a day from the start. A good routine is to do 10 pelvic floor lifts every time the baby is feeding. (Imagine that you are trying to stop a stream of urine after it has started).
- Simple abdominal muscle exercises can be started, just a feeling of tightening the muscles to hold the abdomen in is sufficient.

Two to six weeks

Mothers vary in how quickly they regain their physical tone after childbirth. For some it seems to take no effort and they are back wearing tight jeans within a few weeks. For others it takes much longer, especially if there is has been significant weight gain during pregnancy. Some mothers lose weight rapidly whilst breastfeeding, others do not lose any until they have stopped feeding and then only after a concerted effort. It is a mistake to try to diet in the first few weeks after the birth, especially if trying to get breastfeeding established, because the body has enough to cope with without being deprived of nutrition at this time and dieting may cause the milk supply to suffer. It is more important to undertake regular postnatal exercises to help get the body back into shape.

Most hospitals give new mothers an exercise sheet to help them in the first few weeks. The following exercises are the most important.

- Pelvic floor muscles exercises should be continued many times a day – a guide of 10 pelvic floor lifts every hour. If you can stop your urine flow mid-stream then you are doing well.
- Gradually build up abdominal muscle exercises

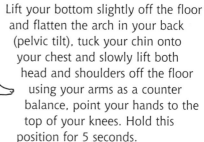

Lift your bottom slightly off the floor and flatten the arch in your back (pelvic tilt), tuck your chin onto your chest and slowly lift both head and shoulders off the floor using your arms as a counter balance, point your hands to the top of your knees. Hold this position for 5 seconds.

Slowly lower yourself to the floor and relax completely.

Repeat 3 times.

In the same position, roll your knees slowly from side to side.

This is good for improving the tone of the abdominal muscles that pull the waistline in.

After six weeks

There should be a gradual return to normal physical activities, it is a good idea to try to undertake some regular form of exercise. There are an increasing number of sports facilities that provide a creche, or that run specific postnatal exercise classes. Whatever your chosen form of exercise, it is much easier to make it a regular part of your life if it is something that you enjoy.

Emotional stress, fatigue and postnatal depression

The intense excitement of the first few days inevitably passes and the daily routine of 24 hour care of the baby and persistent sleep deprivation begins to take its toll. At some point the mother comes down off her 'high', and usually feels exhausted and/or weepy. It is very common to have one particularly weepy day 4 or 5 days after the birth, which is due to hormonal changes.

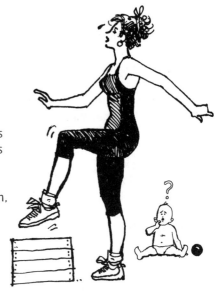

Some mothers take some time to return to feeling 'normal' after the birth. This may be due to physical discomfort from sore stitches, breastfeeding difficulties, headache, fatigue and sleep deprivation, or just not feeling right emotionally. It can be a very confusing time emotionally with highs and lows for no apparent reason. Many mothers are elated when their long awaited baby finally arrives and life continues happily despite a few physical discomforts. For others, even if the baby is very much planned and wanted the mother may feel unaccountably low and depressed in the weeks and months after the birth. She may not feel 'bonded' to the baby, may resent the baby's presence and find adjusting to the demands of her new lifestyle very difficult. This can be the start of postnatal depression.

A new mother will often try to cover up any such emotions, feeling that it must be her own fault, or due to some failing in her as a mother. She may be aspiring to be the perfect mother of her much wanted baby and feel guilty at feeling down and unable to cope. It may be that a close member of the family is the first to notice that there is a problem.

In some cases postnatal depression has a physical cause that is readily treatable osteopathically. During the birth the sacrum can become unseated from its normal position in the pelvis, commonly sagging forwards and down into the pelvis. This position of the sacrum causes tension through the spinal meninges (the very sensitive coverings over the spinal cord) that are continuous with the cranial meninges (the

77

coverings of the brain). This may impose a drag on the brain itself, which can subtly alter the brain chemistry and cause postnatal depression. Treatment to correct the position of the sacrum may have a dramatic effect on the emotional state of the mother.

Even if a mother does not have full postnatal depression, it is common for her to feel that she is just not right in herself. This is often due to the fact that she has physical strains and stresses remaining from the pregnancy and birth, and osteopathic treatment can be of great help.

Family dynamics

The arrival of a new baby has a great impact on the relationship between both parents. The father goes through great emotional changes as well as the mother. For him, it may be a combination of intense love and feeling proud of his new family, but at the same time a realisation of a new level of responsibility for providing for them. He may also feel somewhat excluded or even jealous of the close relationship between the mother and new baby, especially if the mother is breastfeeding. These are all normal feelings.

Fathers can be involved in caring for the new baby by changing nappies, winding and settling the baby after feeds, or coping with crying or colic attacks. If the baby is bottlefed he can obviously help, or can give a breastfed baby a feed of expressed breastmilk. This can work well during the evening to allow the mother to catch a few hours unbroken sleep. Fathers can also play a very important role in making sure that the mother is taking care of herself and eating properly. It is easy to forget or not find time to eat when looking after a young baby.

It is very important that both parents find some time in the day or week to sit down and talk together, so that both can understand how the other is feeling. The old saying that problems shared are problems halved has a lot of sense in it.

Back strain from caring for young children

The first year of a baby's life is physically and emotionally demanding for every parent. As the baby grows and puts on weight, lifting and caring for him/her can place extra strain on the mother's (or father's) back. This extra load is added to any postural strain from the pregnancy or labour which may have left the back vulnerable.

If the baby is fretful and requires carrying around for long periods of time, even a tiny baby can become very heavy and tiring to carry. At this stage the baby does not support his own weight and is often carried on one shoulder. Some mothers (but not all) find that a front sling is an easier way to carry a young baby for long periods of time.

Any task that involves lifting the baby whilst in a leaning forward or twisted position places great strain on the back. This includes bathing and changing the baby, lifting the baby in and out of a cot, and especially lifting car seats in and out of cars.

Carrying a baby or toddler on one hip is second nature to most mothers. Whilst this may be convenient, it places the mother's spine in a very asymmetrical posture and often gives rise to backache. Osteopaths recognise a mother's child-carrying posture as a common cause of back problems.

Self help tips to prevent back strain whilst caring for a young child.
- Whenever possible, keep your back straight and bend your knees to lift the baby.
- For older children, sit down and invite them to come to you for a cuddle without lifting them up.
- Raise the height of the cot base and/or drop the cot side down until the child is able to sit or stand up in the cot.
- For young babies a raised changing surface such as a chest of drawers can minimise the need to bend, but the baby should never be left unsupervised on such a surface even when tiny. As the baby gets more mobile, kneeling down with the baby lying on a bed is often a safer way to change nappies.
- Ideally car seats should not be put into the car with the baby already strapped in, because the combined weight of the baby and the awkward angle of the car overloads the mother's spine.
- Try not to carry a child on one hip for long periods, where possible use alternate hips. Front slings, or backpacks as the child gets older, can be more comfortable and cause less back problems.

7

Treatment of the growing child

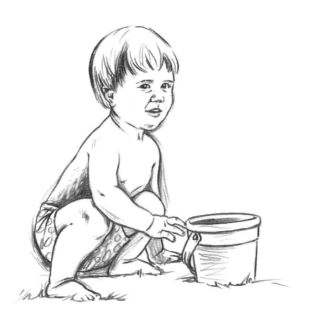

*A*s children grow, they generally grow out of most of the crying, difficulty in sleeping, and feeding etc. that they may have experienced as young babies. However, if the retained moulding is not treated to help it to release, they may begin to suffer secondary effects as they grow. Many of the conditions mentioned in this chapter are very common. Some may be directly caused by the retained moulding, some indirectly. Some children naturally have a better vitality and ability to cope with the retained moulding with minimum effect, others find it much harder and have more obvious signs of it. However, almost all children benefit from osteopathic treatment to release retained compression.

Infections

Many people are surprised to learn that osteopaths treat infections of all sorts. Osteopathic treatment in these cases has a variety of objectives in order to assist the body to fight infections efficiently. Firstly the local area of the infection has to have a good blood supply and free drainage of waste products away from the area. Another particularly important area to work on is the lymphatic system. This is a system of tiny channels that return excess fluid from the periphery of the body back to the venous system. It is within this system that much of the immune response works, the body's way of fighting infections.

The chest area is the key to the lymphatic system. The thymus gland sits just under the sternum or breastbone. This is where many of the cells of the immune system are manufactured. Tension in the upper ribs or trauma to this area can reduce the efficiency of the thymus gland, and also limit the ability of the immune cells to leave the gland and make their way to wherever they are needed in the body.

The main lymphatic channel of the body through which lymph is returned to the venous blood circulation, passes up inside the chest and joins a vein just under the left clavicle (collar bone). If the diaphragm is held in a tense state, or if the ribs are held stiffly and do not move easily with each breath, then this can delay the passage of lymph through the chest. This is a major factor in reducing the ability to fight any infection.

Osteopaths therefore always pay particular attention to the chest area for any infective conditions. Not surprisingly chest infections themselves respond very well to osteopathic treatment, particularly the residual cough and breathlessness that is often left over after an infection (often misdiagnosed as asthma).

In the head, retained birth moulding compression limits the normal formation and drainage of air sinuses in the head, as well as limiting the venous drainage. This can make the child more vulnerable to infections, particularly ear and sinus infections.

Ear infections

Recurrent ear infections in children are so common as to almost be considered normal. In the case of the ear, retained birth compression in the area of the ear is the major contributing factor to recurrent ear infections and glue ear. Children exposed to cigarette smoke are also more likely to develop recurrent ear infections, because the smoke slows down the action of tiny hairs (cilia) lining of the ear, that move mucous and help it to drain.

A common area of the skull to suffer warping and compression is around the temporal bone, which houses the ear. At birth the temporal bone is in three bony parts, separated by cartilage (flexible, like the nose and outer ear). The cartilage allows warping and bending of the bone during the birth. If the stresses are unresolved after birth, the bone will 'set' in its warped shape. This directly affects the drainage of the middle ear to the back of the throat via the Eustachian (auditory) tube, and also reduces blood supply to the ear, and venous drainage away from it.

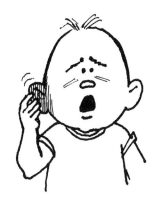

The ear is more likely to become infected when the child has a cold. It does not drain completely afterwards, and is therefore even more vulnerable to the next infection. This situation repeats with infections becoming ever more frequent, until a persistent hearing loss is suffered, and eventually a sticky residue is left in the ear – glue ear.

The auditory or Eustachian tube is a tube that connects the inside of the ear to the back of the throat. It exits from the skull between two bones, and relies on the normal movement between the bones to assist drainage of mucus from the ear. At this point the tube is vulnerable to the effects of restriction of movement between the bones of the skull, such as from retained moulding. If this tube is even partially blocked, then pressure can build up within the ear. The adenoids are lymph glands that sit at the mouth of the Eustachian tube where it drains into the back of the throat. These glands can become enlarged during infections such as colds and block the Eustachian tube, leading to or aggravating ear problems.

Lymphatic drainage from the head is also restricted in cases of retained compression, decreasing the ability to fight infections here.

Ear problems in children respond very well to treatment to reduce the retained birth compression particularly in the region of the temporal bone, to re-establish efficient drainage of the ear, and to improve the function of the auditory tube. The normal response to treatment is of a gradual reduction in the number of ear infections, and an improvement in hearing if this has been a problem. A sure sign of improvement is when a child has a cold that does not result in an ear infection. Severe cases of glue ear may need regular treatment over some months to effect an improvement.

Sinus problems and mouth breathers

Sinuses are air cavities within the bones of the skull. They are invariably made up of two or more bones, and the minute movements between these bones act as a pump to clear excess mucus from the sinuses. If the movement between the bones is restricted for any reason, mucus can build up within the sinuses, causing the nose to become blocked and/or runny.

One of the most common causes of restriction in sinus drainage in children (and adults) is retained moulding compression in the front of the head or behind the eyes. Normal growth and development of the sinuses is impaired, and the normal movement between the bones is restricted. The result is poor development and function of the sinuses. Affected children are often mouth breathers, have a constantly blocked or runny nose, and may find it difficult to blow their nose. The face often looks pinched around the bridge of the nose, and the nose may look unduly small.

The retained compression in the face restricts growth of the middle part of the face – between the eyes and upper teeth. This further restricts function of the sinuses, and may lead to overcrowding of teeth. Orthodontic treatment is often necessary, and the clamping effect around the teeth of wearing a brace can further limit sinus drainage.

For best results these children should be treated before the age of 5 years, when the middle face begins a period of rapid growth. It is usually possible to improve sinus function sufficiently for the child to breathe through the nose. Habitual mouth breathers may continue to breathe through the mouth even after treatment to clear the air passages in the nose. It is important to try to break this habit because it can affect facial and dental development.

Other causes of poor sinus function in both children and adults are direct trauma to the face, from accidents and falls. In older children and adults, dental extractions can traumatise the delicate bones of the face causing or aggravating sinus problems.

If sinus function is mechanically poor, allergies are more likely to develop such as hay fever, or dust allergies. Treatment to improve the mechanical drainage of the sinuses is often successful in reducing the severity of such allergies. Dairy products of all sorts commonly increase the production of mucus, it may be necessary to remove dairy products from the diet in some individuals to help clear a persistent sinus problem.

Behavioural problems and hyperactivity

The pattern started in the early weeks of a fractious baby, poor sleeping pattern and constant need for movement or changes of position, changes as the child grows. These children are uncomfortable when they stay still for too long, and thus are often much happier once they can move around – they often crawl and walk early.

However, their restlessness may lead on to constant fidgeting, difficulty sitting still and concentrating for any length of time, and even to hyperactivity. This often has implications once the child starts school since they find it very difficult to sit still and stay at any one task for more than short periods. This may slow their rate of learning.

Osteopathic treatment often helps the child to calm down, sleep better, sit still for longer periods, and therefore improve concentration and learning.

It may also be important to recognize and eliminate any foodstuffs that may be aggravating hyperactivity. Common foodstuffs which may cause hyperactivity are artificial colourings and flavourings, sugar, chocolate, citrus fruits, potatoes, and wheat.

Learning difficulties

There are many different causes and types of learning difficulties, often similar patterns run in families and have a genetic origin, whilst with others it appears that something specific has happened to the child to cause the problem. A child does not suddenly develop a learning difficulty. The problem has invariably been building up over a period of time, and at some point is identified and given a label. Osteopaths believe that some learning difficulties are caused or aggravated by the accumulative effect of physical stresses and tensions in the body, often the result of a difficult birth. It is also possible for a child to suffer minimal brain damage during birth due to a shortage of oxygen, which may not be apparent at first but may cause some type of learning difficulty later on.

There is a very common pattern of development that precedes an obvious learning difficulty at school. It is interesting to note the similarity of these signs with those of retained birth compression.

• The child often has a history of a difficult birth, was a demanding baby who cried a lot and slept poorly.

- He/she may have reached physical milestones such as sitting crawling and walking early, and liked being on the move. This is generally a response to physical discomfort when staying still that encourages the child to become mobile, and is not necessarily a sign of an 'advanced or intelligent' child.
- As a toddler he/she may have displayed some hyperactive tendencies or have been a 'butterfly' type personality flitting from one thing to the next but not becoming engrossed in one activity for long, so he/she did not learn to concentrate for periods of time.
- The sleep patterns often remains poor, with the child being slow to drop off to sleep and waking easily. Subtle signs of sleep deprivation are irritability and poor concentration.
- The immune system is often depleted, with the child succumbing to many infections. Ear infections are common due to congestion in the ear from retained birth moulding, as well as persistent sinus problems from underdeveloped nasal sinuses, and these children are often mouth breathers.
- After about the age of 7, headaches are common as the bony joints (or sutures) of the skull become fully developed and reduce the overall ability of the skull to cope with any distortion that still persists from birth.
- Once the child is at school, he/she is expected to sit still and focus on one task for extended periods of time. The child often finds this very difficult and so fidgets and is easily distracted.

All these signs are common effects of retained birth moulding. The influence of such strains on normal development cannot be under-estimated.

The first sign of a problem may be that the child does not keep up the expected pace of learning at school, or displays disruptive behaviour due to his/her inability to sit still. In some cases it may be that the child has only been able to keep up with his peers by putting in great effort. Eventually it becomes harder and harder for the child to keep up and a problem becomes apparent. Such a child is often unduly fatigued especially after a day at school.

The earlier a problem is noticed, the better the chances of appropriate help being given in time to prevent a more severe problem developing. The younger a child receives osteopathic treatment to correct physical strains that might contribute to learning problems, the more likely it is to have a significant effect in reducing the degree of the difficulty. It is never too late to treat, although the impact on the learning problem tends to become less as the child gets older. Appropriate treatment at any age can help in improving concentration, and children often seem to grasp new concepts more easily after a course of osteopathic treatment.

The assessment of a child with learning difficulties should include both a learning assessment in which specific approaches to teaching to best help the child can be identified, and a physical assessment which should include sight and hearing tests and an osteopathic assessment. Osteopathic treatment is only one aspect of the treatment and support of a child with learning difficulties, but it can be an extremely valuable one. Osteopaths should be part of a team of support that includes specific teaching such as that given by 'special needs' teachers, which is vital to help to assist the learning process.

The influence of eyesight on learning

The development of good eyesight is a complex process, requiring the eyes to be able to accurately receive images, and the brain to be able to interpret and integrate the information. Any difficulties in any of these areas can have a marked influence on learning, especially once the child gets to school and is required to focus the eyes for extended periods of time.

Physical distortion around the eyes from retained moulding can have a significant effect on eye function. The shape of the eye socket may be altered, and is often different on each side. This may change the acuity – or ability to of the eyes to focus. It may also create undue tension in the eye muscles. The same distortion can impede the venous drainage from the eye, causing sore or dry eyes. Headaches are common especially around and behind the eyes. Osteopathic treatment to correct mechanical strain around the eyes can have a measurable effect on eye function. Osteopaths often liaise with Behavioural Optometrists to find the most appropriate treatment for each child.

Behavioural Optometrists specialise in assessing and treating visual problems in children with learning difficulties. A Behavioural Optometrist assesses not only the visual acuity – or ability of the eyes to focus, but also many aspects of vision including how the brain interprets images. Assessment includes testing the ability of the eyes to track evenly along a line of words as in reading. This is often very difficult for a child, and their eyes may jump about, missing out words and making reading slow and laborious. Treatment may involve prescribing glasses, or vision therapy in which eye exercises are used to train the eyes to work better, and to help the brain integrate sight with other physical aspects of development. The results of such treatment are often dramatic if vision is a major cause of the learning problem, with rapid improvements in many areas including concentration, reading speed and comprehension, and handwriting.

Dyslexia

In addition to all the above general information about the treatment of children with learning difficulties, there are also specific areas of physical tension in the head that can be associated with dyslexia.

Warping or strain in certain areas of the skull can be associated with specific learning difficulties, one such area is in the temporal bone that houses the ear. Mechanical stresses within the temporal bone can result in tension being transmitted to the brain directly underneath it. The brain here is involved in speech and word recognition and this type of compression can interfere with normal development in these areas. It is commonly associated with dyslexia and other learning difficulties.

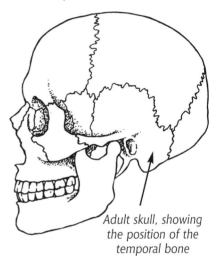

Adult skull, showing the position of the temporal bone

Dyspraxia

Dyspraxia is the name given to a specific difficulty with learning balance and co-ordination of muscles. It may show as difficulties with fine motor skills such as the hand control required in learning to write, or in gross motor skills and balance such as in learning to ride a bike or catch a ball. The child may appear clumsy or fall over a lot.

In order for the muscles to develop the fine control needed to perform physical tasks accurately, the body framework needs to be balanced and stress free, and the brain needs to give the correct messages to the muscles.

For example:

There is a strong relationship between the eyes, ears and posture. The eyes and ears work together to maintain balance, and both need to be held level in order to function properly. Any asymmetry in the posture such as carrying the head on one side, perhaps as a result of a birth-related trauma, is compensated by changes in the shape of the curves throughout the spine. There may be increased tension in the neck and shoulder muscles from the neck strain, but also throughout the whole spine as a result of the body's attempt to keep the eyes and ears level, and maintain balance. This child is at a disadvantage from the start in attempting to learn to control and co-ordinate the muscles of his body and may appear awkward or clumsy, or have poor control of balance. He may be relatively late learning to walk because it takes longer for him to master the necessary co-ordination and balance.

The area of the brain that controls co-ordination is called the cerebellum, and is situated low down inside the back of the skull, in the region of the occipital bone. It is possible for the cerebellum to become slightly pinched or crowded if there is any limitation in the normal slight movement between the bones of the skull in this area (the occiput and temporal bones) or in the junction of the occiput with the top vertebra of the spine. This can impede the development of fine muscle control in any area of the body. Such limitation to bony movement can result from birth trauma, but can also be caused by heavy falls on the back of the head, or sit-down falls on the bottom. A sit-down fall causes the head to impact heavily on the top of the spine, and focuses strain at the base of the skull where it joins the first cervical vertebra of the neck. In the pliable bones of a child this can cause the occipital bone to buckle slightly and crowd the brain underneath, in the region of the cerebellum. Dyspraxia may be the result.

Case History

Jake had received osteopathic treatment soon after birth to release his retained moulding, and responded well, becoming a happy baby who slept well. He was brought in for treatment again when aged 2 years because his sleep pattern had deteriorated, he was waking several times a night and was miserable in the day. When observed playing with toys in the waiting room before his appointment, it was noticed that his movements were awkward, he moved with straight legs especially getting up from sitting into a standing posture, and he walked on tiptoes. He appeared quite dyspraxic.

Jake's sleep and general behaviour had deteriorated following several falls on the back of his head, and although his parents had noticed that he walked on tiptoes they were not unduly worried. This too had been more noticeable recently.

On examination, it appeared that as a result of the recent falls there was marked tension in the top of the neck, with limitation of the normal motion in the back of the skull in the region of the occipital bone. This was felt to be crowding the cerebellum and causing the dyspraxia. Treatment to release these tensions was given.

When Jake was seen again two weeks later his parents reported that he was happy and sleeping well, and he was observed to be moving much more easily and not walking on tiptoes. On examination the tension in the base of the skull and top of the neck had resolved.

Not all children with dyspraxia respond as quickly as Jake did. He had a particularly dramatic response to both the initial trauma of the falls, and then to the release of the effects of the falls, which highlighted the link between the two.

Dyspraxia can be associated with eyesight difficulties. If the eyes do not receive or interpret information accurately, it makes it very difficult for the body to physically respond accurately and quickly, such as in catching a ball. The child therefore appears clumsy. An accurate eyesight test is therefore essential in a child with dyspraxia.

Cerebral palsy and other types of brain damage

If anoxia at birth has been sufficient to cause actual brain damage, it is almost invariably the case that the birth has been difficult, with excessive compressive forces on the baby. The damaged baby is unable to release the moulding and compressive effects unaided, and the treatment of these as already described applies to these children in the same way as any other child.

Osteopathic treatment is unique as a treatment therapy in that it can influence directly the effects of anoxia on the nervous system. This does not mean that osteopathy can 'cure' cerebral palsy, rather that it can help the child develop to the best of his/her potential within the limitations of the brain damage present.

When a child has suffered some brain damage at birth, certain areas of brain tissue have been deprived of oxygen for long enough to cause the death of some cells. Other parts may have sustained temporary damage or small haemorrhages (or bleeds). In addition the brain may swell after a difficult birth, which can cause further damage. On osteopathic examination and treatment the trauma to the brain is palpable, frequently the brain as a whole is felt to be in a state of shock and rigidity, and is unable to express its normal subtle motion. Fluid congestion around areas of damage may also be palpable. These effects can compound the effects of the specific brain damage by imposing restriction to the ongoing development of the healthy areas of the brain. It is a bit like trying to drive a car with the brakes partially on.

Whilst osteopathic treatment cannot repair the areas of cell death in the brain it can help improve overall function of the nervous system, ease congested areas by improving the venous drainage, and assist recovery of the partially damaged areas to their fullest extent. This helps to improve the overall health of the brain thus helping the brain to achieve its maximum potential.

In the daily life of children with cerebral palsy, where the simple things in life are a struggle, any progress is a great achievement. After osteopathic treatment, parents and carers often report small improvements in the health and well being of such children, or the learning of a new skill. They generally become more comfortable and happy.

Febrile convulsions and epilepsy

If a child has a rapid rise in temperature, usually at the start of a fever, it can trigger a febrile convulsion. This is a form of epileptic fit, during which the brain literally short circuits and there is a large electrical discharge. A child should always be checked by a doctor after a fit of any sort.

The shock to the brain of such an event is profound. Immediately afterwards the child may be sleepy, disorientated, and suffer a loss of concentration and co-ordination. The visible recovery may take several days. Osteopathically the effects of a convulsion leave a palpable level of rigidity and shock in the brain. This can render the child more vulnerable to further convulsions, make concentrating difficult, delay development, and aggravate pre-existing problems such as asthma. Specific osteopathic treatment can reduce this shock in the nervous system, and therefore reduce the vulnerability to further febrile convulsions.

Epilepsy is a very complex subject, and each case needs to be assessed individually. In some children (and adults), epilepsy can be reduced by osteopathic treatment. In others, it will not affect the epilepsy itself, but can reduce the ongoing effects of previous fits.

If the epilepsy is severe and uncontrolled by drugs, whilst the child may seem better in him/herself after treatment, i.e. more alert, responsive and happy, the effects are likely to be negated by the next fit.

Headaches, and other aches and pains

Contrary to popular belief, many children do suffer from headaches and musculo-skeletal pain in the same way that adults do. This is hardly surprising since the cause is often the same, namely the retained effects of birth trauma.

Headaches often start in children around the age of 7-8 years, which is when the sutures or joints between the bones of the skull form properly. This reduces the slight pliability of the bony casing of the skull, and so it may be more difficult for the child to tolerate any retained moulding from birth that has left the skull distorted. This may be the first sign of retained compression in the child.

Children may also suffer from growing pains. These are deep-seated aches in the shafts of long bones, usually in the legs, and are generally worse at night. The cause is tension or stress within the bone that is offering resistance to the laying down of new bone as it grows. This may be related to birth, or to the effects of falls and accidents. It is readily treatable osteopathically.

Other musculo-skeletal aches and pains in the body can arise for similar reasons.

Asthma

Asthma is an increasing problem of childhood. There are many different causes, and it varies in severity from a mild cough, or wheeziness after exercise, to a severe and potentially life threatening condition.

There are many different causes of asthma, and it often runs in families. Increasingly pollution and smoking are being recognised as triggers for asthma. Other allergies such as house dust mites, animals and certain foods are relevant in some cases. Stress is another well-known trigger for asthma in vulnerable people. Each case of asthma must be assessed individually. Some cases are amenable to osteopathic treatment, some are not.

Mild asthma may be indicated by delayed recovery from a chest infection. This is often because the strenuous exercise of coughing has caused the muscles and rib articulations of the chest to become very tight and restricted. This prevents the lungs being used to capacity and delays the elimination of retained mucus, resulting in a prolonged cough or feeling of breathlessness on exercise.

Osteopathic treatment of asthma is aimed at improving the function of the chest as far as possible, and at reducing any general body tensions and stresses, such as retained moulding from birth, that may be generally undermining the general health. Overall the aim is to build up a margin of health reserve in the individual so that an asthma attack is not triggered by minor events.

Asthmatic children often exhibit signs of retained birth compression, are often mouth breathers, and may also have suffered some foetal distress (caused by lack of oxygen) during their birth. The control centres for respiration are situated in a part of the brain that is well protected during birth, but they can be affected by the long term effects of compression within the base of the skull. Such compression can reduce the blood flow to this area of the brain very slightly, enough to disturb the normal control of respiration and aggravate an asthmatic tendency.

In asthma the chest itself becomes very stressed due to the increased muscular effort needed to breathe. In more severe cases this alters the development of the rib cage to a classic 'barrel shape'. Most of the respiratory effort is directed to breathing IN, and the ability to breathe OUT is often poor. Treatment to render the rib cage more supple and able to breathe in and out with less effort will often ease a chronic asthmatic state.

Osteopathic treatment may be sufficient to relax the muscles and improve the flexibility of the chest, thus increasing lung capacity. This offers a simple alternative to the use of inhalers. More severe asthma cannot often be eliminated completely using osteopathic treatment, but there is much that can be done to help relieve the effects, and reduce the amount of inhalers necessary.

Dental development

Dental patterns are often genetically determined, and run in families. However, they are also influenced by developmental stresses imposed on the growing face. The same stresses through the base of the skull that limit normal sinus growth and development in children also limit the growth of the face.

This leads to a greater incidence of dental overcrowding, necessitating in some cases dental extractions and orthodontic treatment later on. To prevent this situation as far as possible, treatment of the child is essential as young as possible, but definitely before the age of 5 years. From age

5-10 years the face goes through a period of rapid growth. This needs to progress unimpeded to maximise room for the adult teeth.

Orthodontics

Orthodontic treatment has a dramatic effect on the normal functioning of the face, and can have repercussions throughout the whole body. Consider the effect of placing a clamp around the teeth (the brace), sufficient to cause the teeth to move in their sockets. Normal motion of the facial bones in relation to each other and in relation to the other bones of the head is severely restricted. This demands accommodation by the rest of the head and body. If the overcrowding is as a result of unresolved birth stresses that have restricted growth of the middle face, then the brace adds further compression to an already compromised structure.

During orthodontic treatment it is common for other areas of the body to begin to show symptoms as the body struggles to cope. Headaches, clicking jaws, painful joints particularly the knees, irritability, reduced concentration, neck pain, stomach pains, lowered immunity and an increased vulnerability to musculoskeletal strains are all commonly seen as a direct result of wearing a brace.

Once the brace is removed, the stresses do not always dissipate, and the effects are almost always palpable many years later in adults. There is usually a persistent feeling of pinching and strain through the face and behind the eyes which may cause sinus problems, headaches, or eyestrain. In addition, continuing postural adaptation in the neck may contribute to long term neck or back problems. Not surprisingly osteopaths do not like orthodontic treatment much! However, we do recognise that at times it is necessary, and will do what we can to minimise its effects.

It may not be possible to fully treat a child for other conditions until the brace is removed.

Osteopathic treatment is strongly recommended:

BEFORE the brace is fitted: to reduce the underlying stresses as much as possible
DURING the time the brace is being worn: occasional treatments to help the body accommodate the additional load reduces the secondary symptoms and also helps the teeth to move quicker
AFTER the brace is removed: osteopathic treatment to reduce its long term effects

Development of the spine

Osteopaths are well known for their treatment of spinal related conditions, mainly in adults. Retained moulding in the head from birth can set up stresses through the neck and thus through the rest of the spine that increase the likelihood of back problems in later life.

It is not only the head that can suffer stresses and strains during the birth process. The chest or rib cage is also very vulnerable to twisting and compressive strains as the baby is forced through the narrow pelvis.

One of the many causes of scoliosis (or curvature of the spine) is the stress inflicted on the body and spine of the baby during birth. Osteopathic treatment early in life may not prevent a scoliosis developing, but an osteopath can monitor it and treat when necessary to ensure that the spine is at all times working in a balanced and stress free way. This reduces the likelihood of back problems later in life.

Other problems of childhood

There are many other types of problems in children that are related to birth stresses, and that also respond to osteopathic treatment. This may include the child who is not thriving and eating well, or a child who is just not happy in themselves – they feel 'out of sorts'.

Hormone imbalances

Slow growth in children may sometimes be due to mechanical strain in the region of the pituitary gland. The pituitary gland is a pea sized part of the brain that controls the release of growth hormone. It sits in a bony cradle in the sphenoid bone in the centre of the head, behind the eyes. The gland is richly supplied with blood and relies on the normal slight rocking movement of the sphenoid bone to enable it to function efficiently and release its hormones into the blood stream. This movement can be hindered by the stresses of birth; certain blows to the head, especially to the face; or by the wearing of dental appliances including braces.

It is very common for children to have a growth spurt after a course of osteopathic treatment, part of which is attributed to the improved function of the pituitary gland that controls the release of growth hormone. It may also be partly due to an improved sleep pattern. Most growth occurs whilst we are asleep, so a child who survives on minimal sleep is often small in stature.

In girls, painful, heavy or irregular periods can also be caused by poor pituitary gland function, as well as by tension in the pelvis around the uterus. Falls on the bottom or hips can transmit strain to the ligaments of the uterus causing imbalances or tensions in these ligaments, which then become uncomfortable with the venous congestion of a period. Period problems often improve with osteopathic treatment.

When to seek osteopathic treatment

Children may cope well with their retained moulding compression, and have apparently no problems. However, it may reduce their ability to cope with other trauma in life such as falls, car accidents or emotional traumas.

Children do not need treatment for every minor bump and bruise, but occasionally a child has a particularly nasty fall where perhaps they are stunned or badly shocked. After the fall parents may notice that the child is fractious, or a change in their sleep pattern, or the child may succumb to an infective illness. It is advisable to have the child checked over after such events, to help them fully release the effects.

Falls on the chin are particularly traumatic. They cause a characteristic strain pattern that is poorly accommodated by the body. Many osteopaths will recommend children having occasional treatment as a preventative measure, to address the accumulated effects of accidents and falls that the body has not fully released by itself.

Children can suffer emotional stress just as much as adults. This may be due to tension within the family unit, at school, with peers, bereavement, or for many other reasons. This should always be taken seriously and may need to be taken into account when treating the child. Osteopaths are not trained counsellors, and often cannot change the cause of the stress. However osteopathic treatment may help to alleviate the physical tension generated by emotional stress, and thus help the child cope better.

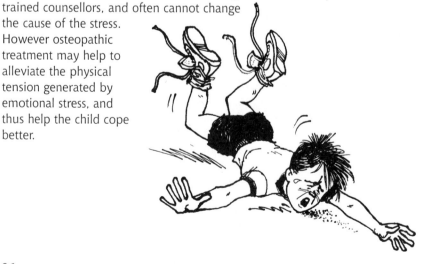

The development of healthy posture

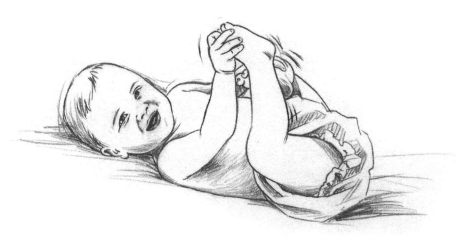

This chapter has been written in association with David Newbound of the Children's Seating Centre.

*B*ack pain has reached almost epidemic levels in the modern world, and more days are lost from work through back pain than any other complaint. Since prevention is better than cure, this chapter is aimed at helping parents understand how to help their children develop good posture, and reduce the chances of developing back problems in later life.

Early reflexes
In a newborn infant, the nervous system is not fully developed. The area of the brain (cerebral cortex) that will eventually allow the child to control his own movements is still forming, and the nerves have not yet developed their myelin sheaths (a kind of insulation around the nerve fibre that assists nerve function). However, the spinal cord is already myelinated and ready

to function at birth, and it is this that controls the newborn's movements. These early movements are all reflex actions, which means that the baby has no control over them, and the movements follow set patterns. Some of these reflex movements are necessary for survival, such as the rooting and suckling reflex, others are precursors to learning to move. The newborn moves legs, arms and body all at the same time.

Once the cortex and myelin sheaths are sufficiently developed the cortex (or voluntary control centre) of the brain gradually overcomes the earlier reflex control of muscles in order to gain voluntary control. This occurs from the top down, so the arms come under voluntary control before the legs. Movements need to be practised many times to lay down a firm pathway of control, and once this is established the child is ready to progress to the next stage.

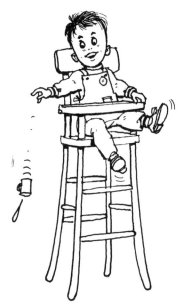

An example of this is the grasp reflex. A newborn baby can grasp a finger placed in his fist very tightly. This is a reflex action at first, but he gradually learns to grasp objects voluntarily as the nervous connections develop. After this, he learns to overcome this reflex in order to be able to voluntarily let go. This is the root of the baby's favourite game of dropping toys onto the floor and waiting for someone to pick them up. This may be a very frustrating process for the parents, but is a very important stage for the child. He is learning how to grasp objects and then let go. He is also learning that he can engage a response from adults, on his terms. Whilst at first the nervous system is not sufficiently mature to allow the baby to control his limbs and body, the sensory nerves are active throughout the body from birth. From the start the brain is receiving a constant barrage of information about the body and limbs, such as where the limbs are in space, the position of the joints etc. This is important information that the brain needs in order to learn control, co-ordination and balance.

The nervous system develops at different rates in different children, and a child will not move on to a new stage until his nervous system, co-ordination and muscle strength are sufficiently developed.

Movement and development of the spine

Head Control

From the earliest days in the uterus, the spine develops as a 'C' shaped curve from top to bottom. As the baby learns to lift his head, learning firstly to turn the head, and then to hold it up, the neck is arched back. This encourages the development of the spinal muscles at the back of the neck and begins the 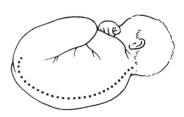 development of the secondary adult 'S' curve of the spine. The muscles of the neck have to develop both strength and co-ordination in order to be able to support and control the head.

This process can be encouraged by allowing the baby to lie on his stomach for short periods each day. Natural curiosity will encourage him to lift his head, and gradually he will develop the strength and control to be able to hold his head up for longer periods. Lying on the front is very important for the baby's development, it straightens the hips, strengthens the back muscles and helps in the development of head control. With the recommendation that babies sleep on their backs as it lowers the risk of Sudden Infant Death, or Cot Death, babies tend to spend less time on their front.

Whilst head control is becoming established, the baby is also learning to control his arms. This begins as a random flailing of the arms, and movements gradually become more controlled and purposeful. The baby learns to roll over first by accident, and then at will. This coincides with learning to suppress another primitive reflex.

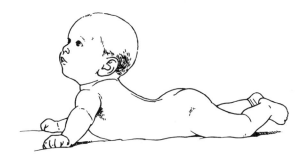

Sitting

In order to be able to sit securely, the child has to develop control over the spinal muscles so that he can maintain balance. Sitting is mastered gradually, the child firstly using the feet to aid balance, and later being able to sit on a flat surface such as the floor. At around six months old, a child can learn to sit using his feet to help balance, if placed in an appropriately fitting chair with a foot support.

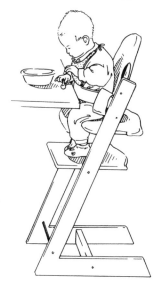

An excellent Scandinavian design of chair called the Tripp Trapp chair is available from the Children's Seating Centre. The special feature of this chair is that it has a fully adjustable seat and foot support so that it grows with the child, and fits babies from 6 months old right through to adults. It allows babies and children to sit comfortably at a table, which is beneficial to them socially and also makes learning manual tasks such as eating and writing easier because their sitting position is stable and balanced.

When a baby of around six months old is placed in such a chair, at first the child's body will flop from side to side in the chair, and then he will begin to explore the foot support, padding with his feet. Gradually in the space of a few minutes the child will learn to use his feet to stabilise his upper body and can sit upright. He is even able to reach for objects beyond his reach at will. This same child placed on the floor will still be unable to sit unsupported.

If a child is made to sit without foot support then the support of the spine has to be more conscious and cannot occur until later (usually 8 months plus). More importantly, a child has no urge to consciously support or balance the spine, so that slumped sitting becomes habitual.

Once the sitting position has been mastered, the baby is able to engage more actively in his environment.

All fours and crawling

As the baby grows and begins to get up onto all fours, and then to crawl, the lower spine or lumbar region is dropped into an extension curve (the normal hollow back). This is a very important stage for the development of the adult 'S' shaped spinal curves, and also for co-ordination of the limbs. The action of crawling involves cross-patterning (using the right arm with the left leg), which is important in suppressing some of the primitive reflexes that a baby is born with. This in turn is an important preparation within the brain for learning other patterns later on.

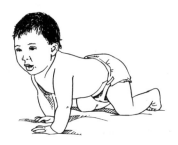

Some children only crawl for a short time, and some master the art of crawling on all fours only after they learn to walk. This is usually sufficient for the suppression of the primitive reflexes. However, many children who have learning difficulties later on are those who never crawled, and therefore did not set up the correct nervous pathways.

Walking

Babies usually develop enough balance and control in the legs for standing and walking between 1 year and 18 months old.

Baby bouncers and sit-in walkers

Babies love being bounced, as every parent knows, and the bouncing helps to stimulate the foot/spine reflexes. An adult bouncing a child will usually get tired and change the child's position regularly, so there is a natural limit to the stress on the baby's back and legs. However, children are often left in baby bouncers and sit-in walkers for long periods of time. This is not good for their development for the following reasons:

- A child who is unable to support himself sitting lacks the muscular strength in the spinal muscles to support the spine for long periods of time. This causes the spine to drop back into the primary 'C' curve, and prevents the normal 'S' curves from developing properly. In addition, the immature intervertebral discs are placed under premature load, which can weaken them and contribute to long term back problems.

• Prematurely placing the child in a sit-in baby walker allows him to be mobile early. This may make him happier because he is more entertained, but it discourages the crawling process, which may be missed out altogether.

Babies should ideally spend most of their day lying flat in varying positions, or in semi-reclining seats (but only for short periods), until they learn to move of their own accord.

The effects of birth stresses on the development of mobility

A baby that is uncomfortable in any part of their body as a result of retained birth stresses will seek to reduce that discomfort. This is the same as in any of us, if we are uncomfortable we will change position. A young baby cannot do this unaided, but quickly finds that crying is a very effective way of getting attention and thus position changes. In the early days, they may prefer being held in particular ways, and like being moved or rocked. As they grow, any discomfort when lying down (such as the pressure of a pillow on a stressed head or neck), gives them incentive to learn to move quickly.

These babies will often be the ones to learn to sit, crawl or walk early. This is not always a sign of an 'advanced child', but may be a natural response to discomfort. Parents often notice how much happier a fractious child becomes when he learns to move around. Contented babies do not have the incentive of discomfort to encourage them to move early, and will learn to move in their own time, often in a more relaxed and controlled fashion.

Osteopathic treatment of babies to release the effects of retained birth stresses is of great benefit in allowing them to learn to move and control their bodies in a relaxed and confident manner. A child will often achieve the next stage of development soon after a treatment. Certainly this applies if they are on the brink of trying to crawl, or walk.

The development of posture

What do we mean by posture?

Many of us grew up constantly being told to 'stand up straight', 'pull your shoulders back', 'stop slouching' and other such instructions, and as a result many people have the impression that good posture is simply the ability to stand or sit up straight with the shoulders held back.

Good posture is much more complex than this. Ideally the body should maintain itself in a constant state of balance as we move, so that minimal muscular effort is required to maintain any position. The shape of the spine, the poise of the head, and the way the arms and legs are carried, is a dynamic and constantly changing state. Our posture should be automatically maintained by reflex changes in muscle tension to maintain this balanced control.

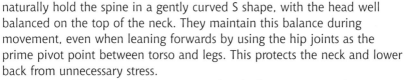

The key here is that minimal muscular effort should be used. If we are using muscular effort to control the position of our shoulders or the shape of our spine, then muscles get into the habit of being tense, which uses up extra energy and we fatigue more easily. We may also suffer from aches and pains as a result of this extra muscle tension.

Young children naturally have well balanced posture with minimal muscular effort. They will naturally hold the spine in a gently curved S shape, with the head well balanced on the top of the neck. They maintain this balance during movement, even when leaning forwards by using the hip joints as the prime pivot point between torso and legs. This protects the neck and lower back from unnecessary stress.

Young children move almost constantly whether sitting, standing or lying down, and even when concentrating there is mobility in the spine, and between the head and neck.

In contrast, older children and teenagers tend to slump in whatever position they are in – standing, lying or sitting. The head is often dropped forwards and sits heavily on the shoulders. The shoulders drop forwards, the rib cage sags down, crowding the heart and lungs inside, and the lower back is often slumped and rounded, especially when sitting. They move much less and look and feel lethargic.

The key point here is that when children maintain 'natural' or 'reflex' control then they intuitively find ways to complete tasks with the head, neck and back relationship maintained. Once they develop bad habits that interfere with natural usage, then neck and lower back take most of the strain, especially in seated positions and lifting. It is easy to see how this can set up long term weaknesses and back problems.

Setting up back problems

Much research has been done on back problems
in children, and most of it makes worrying reading.

One study[11] (Bullock) showed that poor or
awkward posture causes fatigue, strain and
eventually pain. It may result in structural
deformation of the body, pain in the back
and legs, decreased lung capacity, poor
circulation, intravascular pressure, kinks in
the bowel, and many irregularities in the
function of the body.

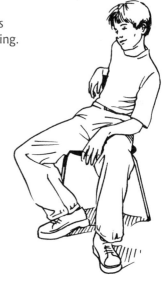

Prolonged sitting in poor positions,
especially during growth spurts, can place
the vertebrae and discs under unnatural
load. A study in 1984[12] (Fisk) showed that
56% of teenage males and 30% of females
suffered from Scheuermann's disease. This is a
softening of the discs and vertebrae which
causes a group of vertebrae to become permanently wedge shaped, with
loss of mobility. It affects the area of the spine just below the lower ribs,
and is a common cause of aching in this region in teenage children.
Frequently there are no symptoms in childhood, but the disease is a strong
predictor of back problems in later life.

Osteopaths are increasingly treating children for back and neck strains
caused by carrying heavy bags. Schools do not always provide lockers for
children, so they have to carry their books around all day. Guidelines from
the National Back Pain Association indicate that children should not carry
more than 20% of their body weight. Many children exceed this on a
regular basis, and in addition carry this weight in bags slung over one
shoulder. Peer pressure is a major problem here, but where possible
children should be encouraged to use a rucksack which spreads the load,
especially for lengthy journeys. The National Back Pain Association sells a
well-designed school bag that is not only comfortable to wear, but spreads
the load over the whole spine and so minimises strain on any one area.
See page 118 for contact address.

What can be done?

We need to ask the question 'why do children lose their natural poise and
balanced posture as they grow'. Whilst low self-esteem and peer pressure

are factors in poor posture, the most significant factor appears to be badly designed furniture.

Modern children spend more time sitting watching TV and playing computer games and less time playing physical games than in the past, so we should look very carefully at the types of furniture they are using and the impact it has on their posture.

Chairs designed for babies and children should provide support for the feet. Most conventional high chairs or children's seats do not have a short enough seat or an adjustable foot support to allow the child to use the feet to aid their balance.

Poor seating in schools and colleges is likely to fatigue the students earlier, leading to a loss of concentration. One of the best investments that any educational establishment could make is to invest in good seating for its students, make lessons shorter and allow more movement time.

Good seating position

A good seating position is one in which the height of the elbows when they are relaxed is at table height, the legs are supported, and the depth of the seat is less than the length of the child's thighs.

For older children and adults, chairs which slope forwards tilt the pelvis into a more natural angle in relation to the spine, discourage slumping in the low back and encourage better posture whilst sitting. It is also helpful to have a writing surface that is sloped to an angle of 12 to 24° this prevents the neck from dropping forwards. Moving chairs and 'kneeling' chairs are also helpful.

Poor seating

Chairs that are too low for the table, too long in the seat or that leave their legs dangling and unsupported, can prevent the natural reflex control of posture, and set up poor postural habits.

- If the seat is too long, the lower back is unsupported and encouraged to slump.

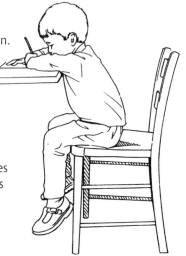

- If the feet are not supported the weight of the lower legs as they dangle presses against the seat front, restricting circulation. The muscles of the spine are reflex-triggered by sensors in the feet. Without foot contact, the spine has to rely more on conscious control.
- If the chair is too low, the child has to raise his arms high and hold them there whilst at the same time trying to learn skills such as eating or drawing. This makes their life difficult, and the learning process hard work – just try it yourself.
- Poor seating will reduce concentration times because of discomfort and fatigue.

Tips for the development of healthy posture:

1 Give young babies a chance to develop neck control and lower back strength by allowing them to progress and develop steadily at their own speed. Make sure they spend time each day lying on their front.

2 Avoid or delay using baby bouncers and sit-in walkers. Children need to develop at their own rate when their body is ready.

3 Baby slings should be of a design that provides support for both the baby's buttocks and thighs, and not be used for extended periods.

4 Try to use chairs (high chairs, carriers, car seats) which have a distinct angle between the base of the thigh and the thighs, these generally offer the spine better support. Gently rounded or curved designs such as hammocks allow the spine to drop into the primary 'C' curve and should only be used for short periods.

5 Make sure that chairs fit the child.

6 Try to ensure that children eat a balanced diet, to encourage healthy bone growth.

7 Once your children are at school age, check that the school allocates right-sized furniture, preferably with sloping desks and no bucket chairs.

8 Don't let them carry a heavy weight on one side. A rucksack is better than a bag, especially for lengthy journeys. Older children should have lockers at school so they do not have to carry their bags all day. For older children who do paper rounds, check their bag weight.

9 Encourage sports and active pastimes. If your children must spend hours in front of a computer, then make sure that they have a good chair, at least with a sloping seat. Chairs that rock can be helpful to keep their muscles active.

10 If you are dismayed to see your child sitting like a sack of potatoes, don't despair, but do take it seriously. It may need someone skilled to help them to want to change. Between 13 and 16 you may find that peer pressure is too great; if so, bide your time unless they report pain, in which case at the very least get them sitting on a wedge of foam and writing at a slope.

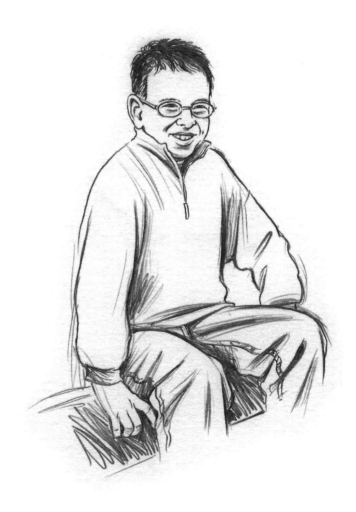

9
Case Histories

❶ JAMES – age 5 months

James had suffered three severe chest infections requiring antibiotics since he was 6 weeks old. Between infections he often sounded tight and congested in the chest. James was a very active baby and generally happy, although he demanded a lot of attention. He slept very little in the day, and woke several times in the night, but was easy to settle again. James was rather a sicky baby, although this was improving since he had been on a more solid diet.

Birth history

James was a first child, and had a long and difficult 27 hour labour. He was a posterior presentation. His mother was given an epidural, and syntocinon to accelerate contractions as her cervix was not dilating well. James eventually became distressed. Both forceps and ventouse deliveries were attempted, but failed. James was finally delivered by emergency caesarean section.

Osteopathic examination and treatment

On examination, James was found to have a very compressed head, with much retained moulding, particularly in the region behind his right ear. This was sufficient to irritate the nerve to the stomach, and cause the vomiting.

In his chest area, the lower ribs were held in a position of exhalation and the upper ribs in an inhalation position, with poor mobility of the ribs during respiration. There was increased muscle tension in the chest area.

After the first treatment James was much happier in himself, slept better, and vomited less. After the second treatment James caught a cold but it did not go to his chest. Three more treatments were necessary to fully release the stresses of birth.

Comment

James' tendency to be sick between feeds was attributed to two factors. Firstly the retained moulding compression within the skull was sufficient to irritate the nerve to the stomach as it exits from the skull. Secondly, stress and distortion through the diaphragm from the repeated coughing made the sphincter into the stomach less efficient.

On examination it was clear that after delivery James had not taken a good 'first breath' to fully expand the lungs, and thus he had not established a good breathing pattern. This increased his vulnerability to chest infections, and made it difficult to fully recover after infections.

❷ GEORGE – age 22 months

George had never slept through the night. His mother reported that George was a happy child in the day, liking to be on the move. He went to bed happily in the evening, but woke several times during the night, and then was difficult to settle back to sleep. He was disturbed by the slightest noise. This had been the pattern since birth.

Birth history

George was born after a 19 hour labour. The second stage (pushing stage) was long and difficult, and George's delivery was assisted by ventouse (suction cup on the head). During the first week, George found breastfeeding difficult, and was very unsettled, sleeping only for short periods. He preferred being carried to lying down.

Osteopathic examination and treatment

Examination revealed that George was suffering a lot of stress from his birth. There was retained compression and distortion within the bony skull, and the top of the neck was twisted and stressed from the delivery. The meninges (coverings around the brain) were in an irritable and hypersensitive state.

Appropriate osteopathic treatment to release the above strains was given. A week later, George returned for his second treatment. His mother reported that his sleep pattern had gradually improved throughout the week. George was given two further treatments to fully release his retained birth stresses, by which time he was sleeping well.

Comment

From George's point of view, the second stage of labour – the delivery part, was highly stressful. His head was squashed and stuck, with very strong contractions bearing down on him. This caused the strain palpable in his head and neck nearly two years later, and was sufficient to make him uncomfortable when lying down and remaining still.

In addition, the ventouse (suction) delivery imposed a strong pull through the membranes on the outside of his head, which are intimately linked to the meninges on the inside. This left the meninges in a shocked and irritable state, and kept his brain in a constantly alert state – so he never went into a really deep sleep.

❸ HANNAH – age 4 years

Hannah had a history of repeated ear infections, and was now suffering from glue ear and deafness.

Birth history

Hannah was a second child. The labour progressed uneventfully, although Hannah was showing some signs of distress. When she was born, she had the cord tightly wrapped around her neck. It was cut after the head was delivered, but it was still some time before her body was delivered, and she took some time to take her first breath.

Osteopathic examination and treatment

Hannah had a moderate degree of retained moulding in her head from birth. In addition the central nervous system (brain) was palpably still in a state of shock, and expressing poor motility (its normal movement) from the hypoxic state suffered during birth.

Hannah was treated 7 times. There was a slow but steady improvement in her hearing, but she still had two further ear infections during this time. After the sixth treatment she had a hearing test, and it was discovered that her hearing was within the normal range. She had no more ear infections after the course of treatment ended.

Comment

The retained moulding compression around the temporal bone (which houses the ear), restricted normal movement within and around the bone. This prevented good fluid drainage from the ear after infection, leaving the ear congested between infections and more vulnerable to the next one.

Restoration of the mobility of the bone was sufficient to clear remaining congestion in the ear, allowing the hearing to return to normal, and removing the vulnerability to further infections.

---

❹ MATTHEW – age 9 years

Matthew had learning difficulties, particularly with reading. He was a highly-strung child, had poor concentration, constant fidgeting and was rather clumsy. He was also a mouth breather, and suffered from asthma, which was controlled by a ventolin inhaler. Matthew complained of frequent headaches. Matthew wore glasses for short sight, and had problems with focusing his eyes.

As a baby he had cried constantly and was a poor sleeper. He had a history of ear infections when younger, but had grown out of these.

Birth history

Matthew's labour was induced as he was overdue. Labour was very strong right from the start, and lasted 11 hours. Matthew's mother had an epidural for pain relief. Matthew showed signs of distress for most of the labour, severe at times. He was delivered using forceps, and had cuts and bruising on his face afterwards.

Osteopathic examination and treatment

Matthew had severe retained compression particularly around his eyes and behind his nose. He had the classic pinched appearance across the bridge of his nose that indicates restricted growth through this part of his face. This caused him to be a mouth breather and also placed strain on the eye muscles, aggravating his eyesight difficulties.

Matthew was treated 8 times during a six month period. There was a gradual improvement in many areas during this time. His headaches disappeared, concentration improved (although he was still very easily distracted), and he seemed much more settled and happier in himself. Comments from his teachers indicated that he was achieving better at school.

Comment

Matthew had to cope with extreme physical compression during labour, particularly when forceps were used to aid delivery. The forceps were necessary because of the degree of distress and anoxia that he was suffering, and as such were possibly life-saving.

A traumatic labour such as Matthew's leaves the head very compressed, and the nervous system in a state of shock. The body is unable to release these effects unaided. As a result Matthew was physically uncomfortable and restless. Normal development of the nervous system was impaired for several reasons: The effects of anoxia during birth leaving a shocked and static nervous system. In addition the ongoing effects of a compressed and rigid container (the skull) limits recovery and development of the brain.

ALEX'S STORY

Alex, my first child, was born after a 40-hour labour. My waters had broken so I had to report to the hospital. I had painful and frequent contractions, but due to a scoliosis in my lower back, his spine jammed against mine, so he got stuck and my cervix didn't open. That night I was given pethidine so I could rest. The following day I received pethidine, and in the afternoon was taken to the delivery suite and given an epidural. I spent over an hour in the second stage of labour, during which time Alex went into distress. When he was born he was

slightly jaundiced, and his head was so misshapen I called him Spud-U-Like.
Breastfeeding was a nightmare. In hindsight his head must have been extremely
painful, and being held to feed must have hurt. He didn't like closeness or being
held much, but so clearly needed contact. He suffered dreadful colic, and used
to kick his legs so hard during an attack, that he kicked one of his toenails off
inside his babygro. Nothing I did seemed to comfort him, so I tried getting him
to suck his thumb. He chewed his thumbnail off. So I reverted to dummies,
which he used to chew into pieces but at least it helped. I gave up breastfeeding
him at three months because it was always so traumatic, and he was much
happier on a bottle. This distressed me. A child who rejected cuddles, and
breast, and contact. According to the usual medical checks and measurements
his physical development continued fairly normally. He crawled before walking
at thirteen months, and talked at about 18 months. But I felt something was
wrong. Part of him always seemed distant and unreachable.

When he started to have tantrums, I noticed a behavioural pattern emerging.
First he would get frustrated by something or someone, and then when the
frustration reached a certain point something else would click in, and the
tantrum would begin. Firstly he would use his head like a battering ram,
growling and charging head first, banging into things, eventually pushing
himself into a cushion in the corner of the sofa. Then he would make a sort of
frustrated, strangled, choking noise, and grip his arms tightly by his sides
flapping his hands like flippers. His legs would be kicking. He would sweat
profusely with the effort, and go red in the face. Sometimes he would shout 'I'm
stuck, I'm stuck'. It dawned on me that part of him was still psychologically
stuck in the birth canal, and couldn't get out. But I realised that he had made it
out and had nothing to fear. So I started holding his head and drawing my
hands round it to give the feeling he was emerging headfirst. This used to calm
him, but the implications worried me.

As Alex grew older he developed a tendency to withdraw completely into
certain solitary activities, and would throw a tantrum if interrupted. When he
was three and a half, a homoeopath noticed his behaviour and gave him a
remedy to help. But in homoeopathy the condition can get worse before it gets
better. He withdrew completely from everyone around, and threw a massive
tantrum and screamed he was stuck when I tried to put him into his car seat.
That night he awoke screaming with frustration and pain. When I tried to
comfort him he demanded to be left alone in the dark in his bedroom with the
door closed. I refused but respected the personal space of his bed. He kept this
tantrum up for about three hours. Eventually he fell into an exhausted sleep.
The following day he had no voice, but the tantrums and withdrawal continued
through the week and gradually became less severe. Since that horrific week he

has refused to sleep with the door closed, and has somehow seemed much more present, acknowledging the world and people around him. I sometimes wonder if he was on the verge of autism because of his birth experience.

Then the physical problems started. Firstly on his first trip to the dentist I was told he had a cross bite, which meant that his top and bottom jaws met asymmetrically affecting the way his teeth fitted together. The dentist blamed it on the fact that I had given him a dummy. Next, he was diagnosed as having poor hearing due to glue ear, and was monitored by the city hospital. He received no treatment however. Then I noticed that when he ran, he put in lots of effort but had such poor co-ordination and balance that he was all over the place, and his efforts were wasted.

Then a friend sent me a booklet on cranial osteopathy, and I decided that I had to get Alex checked out at least. By this time he was six years old. The cranial osteopath told me that he was indeed badly affected from his birth experience. The homoeopathy had helped with the emotional legacy, but the physical legacy still remained which meant that the emotional component might still be triggered. Physically Alex was in a bad way, with his head and body remaining severely compressed and traumatised from the birth. The cranial osteopath imperceptibly manipulated his head and spine, which Alex seemed to enjoy. His glue ear cleared up within months. He still has a cross bite, although it is not as bad as it was, and now his head is growing and he is getting his adult teeth, it is a good time to address this problem. It seems the top half of his skull is contorted in one direction and the lower half and jaw contorts in the other direction. His posture had improved and he is much more efficient in body co-ordination now. He even won one of the running races on school sports day.

Alex is now eight years old, and has been receiving regular cranial osteopathy. The emotional scars although much less, still remain. He enjoys a good cuddle these days and generally he is an outgoing bright little boy, chatty and attention seeking. However, at times of stress he withdraws into that unreachable place, and if he gets very frustrated he occasionally reverts to 'stuck' behaviour. Sitting on the London Underground recently, the train stopped between stations and he confided in me that getting stuck in the Tube with all the lights off would be his worst nightmare. I could see what he meant.

I now recommend all my friends to take their new-borns for cranial osteopathy as soon as possible, and where possible I arrange for a session as my gift to the new baby. If only I had known about cranial osteopathy when he was younger, so much pain could have been avoided, and his babyhood would have been so much happier. I wouldn't want any child to go through such unnecessary physical and emotional suffering as Alex has done, and look forward to the time when all new-borns are routinely checked by a cranial osteopath.

10

Osteopathic Examination and Treatment

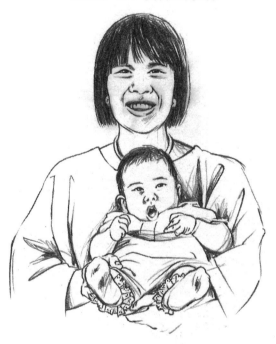

Case history, examination and treatment

At the first visit to an osteopath, a full and careful case history is taken, including detail about the pregnancy, labour and delivery, any illnesses, accidents or notable events in the child's life. This is followed a detailed osteopathic examination and treatment.

The treatment is often so gentle that it may appear that the osteopath is doing nothing more than placing their hands on the child. In reality a great variety of very complex treatment approaches and techniques are being used.

A treatment will usually include some period of palpatory 'observation' by the osteopath, while he/she is assessing the stresses and strains within the baby or child. In addition, specific manipulative techniques may be employed, sometimes very gentle and at other times quite firm.

The chosen treatment approach is applied to the baby or child where necessary to enable the inherent healing ability of the body to effect the release of stresses.

Children generally enjoy their treatment, and often fall asleep during it. However, if compression and stress in the body are extreme, the build up to the release during treatment may be uncomfortable to the child as it focuses them on their 'stressed' areas. This is a temporary situation and soon passes, leaving the child relaxed.

Does the child need to lie still during treatment?

Children are naturally inquisitive and active, and it is a lot to ask a child under 5 years old to lie still during a treatment. Osteopaths become very good at treating children 'on the move', and the position of the child during treatment is very flexible.

Young babies can be treated while they are breast or bottle feeding, which often makes for a quieter life! From 6 months to 4 years, any approach that works is used. Many osteopaths have an array of toys, books and story tapes to amuse the children during treatment. Most children over 5 years old will lie down and listen to stories, or a story tape.

Parents and carers should come prepared to entertain the child in order that the osteopath can concentrate on the treatment.

Preparing a child for treatment

Children are naturally anxious about new experiences, including seeing an osteopath for the first time. Their parents or carers can help to make the experience a happy and relaxing one by following a few simple guidelines:

- It is helpful for the family to arrive in good time for their appointment, so that they can relax and settle in before the treatment.
- Children should be told beforehand who they are seeing and why, and that the osteopath will be touching different parts of their body. Some children are reluctant to be touched, but it is rare to come across a child that cannot be distracted and the treatment to proceed without their really noticing it.
- Bring favourite toys, books or tapes. Older children usually enjoy new toys and books, younger ones may like the security of the familiar.

Could there be any adverse reactions?

Response to treatment is individual and variable. Usually children are calm and happy after treatment, and symptoms gradually settle over a few days. They are sometimes very tired, as their body's energy is redirected towards the healing process. On occasions children have a burst of energy afterwards, as they enjoy the release of tensions and stresses in their bodies.

Occasionally children are unsettled after treatment, this is usually when the release of the retained compression has been incomplete. It is not always possible for them to release it all in one session, especially if the compression is severe. These reactions are only temporary.

How many treatments will be needed?

This is variable, but for a baby the average number of treatments is three to six. This varies according to the severity of the problem.

When to treat

The best time to treat babies is within a few days of their birth. This is when the un-moulding process is naturally at its most active. It is never too soon to treat a baby.

The effects of birth stresses are best treated as young as possible, as the longer they have been there, the longer it takes for the body to release them. However, there is much that can be done particularly under the age of 5 years.

As osteopaths we often need to treat the effects of retained birth compression in our adult patients, so it is never too late to treat.

The treatment of babies after birth is of paramount importance in practising preventative medicine and can help both mother and baby recover from one of the most demanding experiences of their lives.

Do all osteopaths treat children?

Most osteopaths treat children for spinal related problems, and such things as joint strains, using traditional techniques.

However, the concepts described in this book are embraced by the cranial approach to osteopathy. There are a growing number of osteopaths who use the cranial approach and specialise in the treatment of children.

If you are not sure whether your local osteopath treats children, it may be a good idea to talk to him/her before booking an appointment to discuss whether he thinks that he could help your child.

How to find an osteopath

At present there is no separate designation within the Register of Osteopaths indicating practitioners specialising in the treatment of children using cranial techniques. The following organisations will be able to refer you to your nearest:

Osteopathic Information Service
Osteopathy House, 176 Tower Bridge Road, London SE1 3LU
Tel: 020 7357 6655
Website: www.osteopathy.org.uk

The Osteopathic Centre for Children
109 Harley Street, London W1N 1DG
Tel: 0207 486 6160

Useful Addresses

The British Association of Behavioural Optometrists
The Secretary
BABO
72 High Street
Billericay
Essex
Website: www.behaviouraloptometry.com

Children's Seating Centres
3 Quoiting Square, Oxford Road, Marlow, Bucks, SL7 2NH
Tel: 01628 477100

11 Whitcomb St., London WC1A 7HA
Tel: 0207 930 8308

National Back Pain Association
The NBPA have produced well-designed rucksacks that minimise strain on the spine. Contact address:
Wave Express Ltd
7 Atlas Business Centre, Oxgate Lane, London NW2 7HJ
Tel: 0208 450 4549

References

1 *Human Embryology*. William J. Larsen. Pub. Churchill Livingstone.
2 *Psychosocial Predisposing Factors in Infantile Colic*. Rautava, Helenius and Lehtonen. British Medical Journal. Vol 307. September 1993.
3 *Osteopathy in the Cranial Field*. H. Magoun. Pub. Sutherland Cranial Teaching Foundation 1976.
4 *Infantile Colic – Seasonal Incidence and Crying Profiles*. Lehtonen, Liisa. Korvenranta, ki. Archives Paediatric Adolescent Medicine1995. p149 533 – 536.
5 *Infantile Colic: occurrence and risk factors*. Stahlberg MR. Eur J Pediatr 1984;143:108-11.
6 *Parental diary of Infant and Fuss Behaviour*. Barr R.G, Kramer M.S, Boisjoly C, McVey-White L., and Pless I.B. Archives of Disease in Childhood, 1988.
7 *Prevalence of Infant Colic*. Hide and Guyer. February 1982. Archives of Disease in Childhood 1982 p559 – 560.
8 *Charting infant distress: An aid to defining colic*. Hill, FRACP, Menahem, MD FRACP, Hudson, MSc, PhD. Sheffield, MSc, FRACP, et al. The Journal of Paediatrics, Vol.121 No. 5, Part 1, November 1992 755-758.
9 *Infantile Colic: Association with Lactose and Milk Intolerance*. W.M. Liebman MD, JAMA, Feb 20, 1981 – Vol 245, No. 7.
10 *Infantile Colic: The effects of Cranial Osteopathic Treatment on the Behavioural Patterns of Affected Infants*. Clive Hayden, 1996. Paper awaiting publication.
11 *Bullock*, Physiotherapist 1990
12 *Fisk* 1984